AF901936

Psychology Revivals

Telepathy and Medical Psychology

First published in 1947, the original blurb for *Telepathy and Medical Psychology* reads: 'An increasing mass of evidence compiled during the past years has made the occurrence of telepathy and related phenomena an established fact. However, contemporary medical psychology has refused so far to acknowledge their existence and to reconcile them with their systems of thought. Dr Ehrenwald's book is the first serious attempt in this direction. He shows that telepathy is subject to much the same psychological laws as govern dreams, neurotic symptoms and certain manifestations of mental disease. His approach moves largely along the lines of the psychoanalyst, but his conclusions are likely to shake some of the basic propositions of psychoanalysis itself. At the same time they throw fresh light on certain aberrations of character and personality and his new interpretation of paranoia and related disorders may well mark a turning point in modern psychopathology and psychiatry.

Dr Ehrenwald writes his book not only for the medical psychologist: the problems discussed called for the attention of a wider public and his way of presentation makes it fascinating reading for the educated layman.' Today it can be read in its historical context.

Telepathy and Medical Psychology

Jan Ehrenwald

Routledge
Taylor & Francis Group
LONDON AND NEW YORK

First published in 1947
by George Allen & Unwin Ltd

This edition first published in 2025 by Routledge
4 Park Square, Milton Park, Abingdon, Oxon, OX14 4RN

and by Routledge
605 Third Avenue, New York, NY 10017

Routledge is an imprint of the Taylor & Francis Group, an informa business

© 1947 Jan Ehrenwald

All rights reserved. No part of this book may be reprinted or reproduced or utilised in any form or by any electronic, mechanical, or other means, now known or hereafter invented, including photocopying and recording, or in any information storage or retrieval system, without permission in writing from the publishers.

Publisher's Note
The publisher has gone to great lengths to ensure the quality of this reprint but points out that some imperfections in the original copies may be apparent.

Disclaimer
The publisher has made every effort to trace copyright holders and welcomes correspondence from those they have been unable to contact.

A Library of Congress record exists under LCCN: 48013256

ISBN: 978-1-032-95323-6 (hbk)
ISBN: 978-1-003-58434-6 (ebk)
ISBN: 978-1-032-95328-1 (pbk)

Book DOI 10.4324/9781003584346

TELEPATHY AND MEDICAL PSYCHOLOGY

BY

JAN EHRENWALD

M.D. (New York)

Formerly Assistant Physician, Departments of Neurology and Psychiatry, Universities of Prague and Vienna; formerly Acting Medical Officer, The Royal Western Counties Institution, Starcross; Fellow of the Royal Society of Medicine; Member of the Society for Psychical Research; Corresponding Member of the Inter-Allied Health Charter Study Group, etc.

WITH AN

INTRODUCTION

BY

GARDNER MURPHY

LONDON

GEORGE ALLEN & UNWIN LTD

FIRST PUBLISHED IN 1947

All rights reserved

PRINTED IN GREAT BRITAIN
in 11-point Baskerville type
AT THE UNIVERSITY PRESS
ABERDEEN

Preface

PROFESSOR McDOUGALL, in his Foreword to J. B. Rhine's book on Extra-Sensory Perception, pointed out that whoever wants to expound his views on matters of psychical research would be best advised first to state his credentials. Mine are twenty years work in the field of neuro-psychiatry and psychotherapy. My professional duties are concerned with hard facts and leave no room for adventures in lofty speculations. I have no occultistic leanings and my contact with mediums or professional " psychics " has been largely confined to interviews and consultations in clinic or consulting room.

My first acquaintance with the problem of so-called paranormal cognition came through a book published by F. von Neureiter, then Professor of Forensic Medicine at the University of Riga, which reported on the case of a feeble minded child, aged nine, in whom a peculiar telepathic reading ability was observed. I gathered from his statement that the child, in addition to being feeble minded, suffered from a special reading disability, so-called congenital word blindness. At that time I was engaged in an investigation of the pathology of alexia, or word blindness, from a neurological point of view, and I commented, in a paper which appeared in a German journal for neurology, on the striking correspondence between a specific defect and a hyper-function of an admittedly unusual kind which seemed to exist in Neureiter's case. Apart from a few somewhat acrimonious remarks by sceptical colleagues who were not prepared to take the evidence presented in Neureiter's report for granted, the paper passed unnoticed in the professional world, as did Neureiter's publication.

It was only following my arrival in this country that I became conversant with the vast amount of work which had been devoted to the same problem by amateur investigators and, in more recent years, by professional scientists both here and in the U.S.A. Neureiter's case was only one among countless equally intriguing observations although they, too, had largely failed to attract the attention of the medical profession. But further preoccupation with the matter convinced me that it is neither the few spectacular occurrences reported in the literature of psychical research, nor the imposing array of statistical data furnished by laboratory experiments, which form the main interest from the medico-psychological point of view.

I was impressed by the increasing weight of evidence of telepathic occurrences which can be observed in everyday life, in dreams, in the psychoanalytic situation, in neuroses and psychoses, if only we are prepared to meet them with an open mind and to surmount our ingrained prejudice against the very possibility of their occurrence. Indeed, a strange reluctance on the part of modern man to accept certain facts—even though their reality can be established beyond any possibility of doubt—is itself a psychological symptom calling for inquiry, and we shall see that its proper appreciation throws light upon the working of our mind and upon certain features of human personality, so far unexplored.

Nevertheless—or rather for this very reason—I have no illusion as to the misgivings which an investigation devoted to such an unorthodox issue is likely to entail. It may be argued that the evidence upon which it is based is too flimsy to carry conviction; that the method applied is ambiguous; that the interpretations suggested are equivocal and the conclusions reached are in flagrant contradiction to our recognised body of experience. Even if this be true it would only call for adducing of more and more convincing evidence, if this be possible, for interpretations which are in accord with a yet greater volume of observational material; and as for the inconsistency of the conclusions drawn with our familiar world picture, this can more appropriately be adjusted by a determined stroke ripping through the old canvas, than by disregarding, or pitchforking out of existence, facts which are at variance with its traditional design.

It is true that the present inquiry has been so restricted in scope that it does not by itself warrant such far-reaching conclusions. It is confined to the problem of telepathy only which, for obvious reasons, is bound to attract the prevailing attention of the medical psychologist, and it leaves the question of alleged clairvoyance, of so-called physical phenomena, etc., outside its frame of reference. Moreover, it is limited to an exclusively medico-psychological approach and does not encroach upon the territory of the philosopher. But the relevance to wider issues of contemporary psychology and science of the argument pursued here goes without saying, even though it will be for others, more competent than the present writer, to comment on these points.

It is customary to conclude the preface to a book with acknowledgments to those who have assisted the writer with their advice and encouragement. In the present case the list is short. Besides my wife who never tired in the tedious task of typing and re-typing its chapters, written in a language foreign to me a few years ago, and besides a few friends and associates whose criticism helped to mature my views, the list includes thanks for the hospitality found in the spiritual climate of this country—and of the U.S.A.—which, in spite of adversities, made the completion of this book possible. I am also indebted to Mr. S. G. Soal, Mrs. K. M. Goldney and Mr. D. West of the London Society for Psychical Research, and to Mrs. L. A. Dale of the American Society for Psychical Research for valuable suggestions regarding the English presentation and for proof reading.

J. E.

Contents

Introduction

In this period of rapid progress both in medical psychology and in the experimental study of telepathy, the thoughtful reader will eagerly greet every serious effort to build a bridge from the one to the other. Sigmund Freud, dominant figure in the medical psychology of this century, confronted the problem of telepathy, and made characteristic incisive comments upon it, but was not prepared to make the radical adjustments in psychoanalysis which would be required should telepathy prove to be an inescapable reality. Psychical researchers, on the other hand, have been rather slow in pressing into service the methods and data of medical psychology, so that telepathy and related phenomena stand in the experimental records like foreign bodies, which the medical as well as the psychological public can neither assimilate, nor indeed, recognise. There is consequently a deep ignorance on the part of psychoanalysts and other medical psychologists regarding contemporary studies in psychical research, while among the psychical researchers there is very limited technical understanding of the positive contributions of depth psychology to the progress of their investigations. Between the two flickering lights there is a great darkness.

Into this darkness Dr. Ehrenwald's book throws new illumination. From a long experience in psychiatry on the continent and in Britain, and from a firsthand acquaintance with the phenomena and the personalities which characterise modern psychical research, he has formulated a series of psychological hypotheses about the nature of the telepathic process. After reviewing the various classes of experimental research on telepathy, he turns to the clinical understanding of the personal dynamics of telepathic communication, with emphasis upon unconscious needs, projective mechanisms, and the devices by which the dream and the waking course of associations find a way to weave the telepathic impressions into the structure of thought. Of special interest and importance is Dr. Ehrenwald's systematic development of the conception of compensation for a biological defect, a "minus function" which leads to the unfolding of a paranormal capacity in the form of telepathic powers.

Not being content with the general description of unconscious dynamics in the telepathic field, Dr. Ehrenwald proceeds to the analysis of various specific mental anomalies and disorders, showing their possible relations to the paranormal, and concluding with two ingenious case studies of individuals who have exceptional telepathic gifts. Thus he gives us not only the explorer's equipment for the invasion of new territory, but a series of maps which suggest the nature of the terrain.

Such a book will be of interest to the alert phsyician, and also to psychologists and to biologists who are not afraid of explorations off the beaten track; and it will prove stimulating to a wider circle of readers who have wondered how and when psychological science will begin to make a serious effort to clarify and to explain the almost uncharted area of telepathic phenomena.

GARDNER MURPHY.

PART I

OUTLINE OF A WORKING HYPOTHESIS

Chapter I

TELEPATHY AND PRIMITIVE MENTALITY

THE time honoured custom of commencing a book with scholarly references to what the ancient Greeks, Romans or Egyptians had to say about its subject-matter can hardly be applied to the problem of telepathy. They may, or may not, have been conversant with what is now meant by thought reading or thought transference, but the term itself is modern and was coined by F. W. H. Myers in 1883.

Telepathy means the perception by a person of another person's mental processes, without the aid of sensory channels. It is usually distinguished from other forms of extra-sensory perception (J. B. Rhine) or psi-phenomena (R. H. Thouless) such as clairvoyance, that is, paranormal knowledge of physical events, alleged precognitive telepathy, or foreknowledge of future happenings, mental or physical, and the like.

However this may be, ancient tradition and primitive belief has been little concerned with these subtle distinctions made by modern psychical research. Indeed, primitive man failed to draw a clear-cut demarcation line between the data of his ordinary sensory experience and the world of his day-dreams and phantasies.

Even to the savage of our days it is by no means more remarkable that a witch doctor is able to bewitch his cow, or to kill his neighbour's wife by his magic than that his son can slay a bird with a stone. To him, the natural and the supernatural imperceptibly merge into one another; they are governed by identical laws and are equally amenable to control by his actions as to the magic power of his incantations. He is convinced that he is able to cause crops to grow, rain to fall, storms to subside, through his rites and ceremonies. He believes that he can cause the death of a foe by performing dismal practices with his effigy, and that his enemy can retaliate on himself in exactly the same way. Indeed, he maintains that whatever he may do, think or desire at any given moment may influence the thoughts, emotions or actions of his fellow-men at a distance.

Accordingly his whole conduct, his tribal customs and his moral code are so designed as to make due allowance for this basic fact of what James Frazer termed telepathic or sympathetic magic. In his *Golden Bough*, he describes scores of examples illustrating this point.

While the Gilyak hunter is pursuing game in the forest, his children at home are forbidden to make drawings on wood or sand " for fear that if they did so, the paths in the forest would become as perplexed as the lines in the drawings so that the hunter might lose his way in the forest and never return ".

A similar tabu is reported about the Dajak wives ; while their husbands are away on a hunting expedition, they are forbidden to touch greasy substances " lest their prey should slip through the fingers of the successful hunter ".

Hottentot women, whose husbands are hunting, have to do one of two things during their absence ; either to light the fire and keep it burning until they come back or go to the water and continue to splash it. If they fail to carry out one of these obligations they believe their men folk would meet with disaster.

The tasks assigned to the Hayda women when their husbands take to the war-path are of a somewhat more pleasing nature, they are asked to dance and sing battle songs, and to arrange everything about them in a certain order. It was thought that the wife could kill her husband if she did not observe these customs.

Various malignant practices of so-called " Black Magic ", connected with the death bone, the magic image, etc., are a familiar feature of primitive belief and have been preserved up to our day.

The witch doctor—who figures so largely in the legends connected with primitive man—makes a figure of clay to represent his foe, strikes a thorn into the place where he thinks his heart to be, and imagines he is able to kill him in this way. Malinovski gave a vivid account of how he would turn and twist his weapon in the air in a state of increasing fury and excitement as if he were actually stabbing his enemy. Such practices are far from being indifferent to the persons against whom they are directed. " If the victim gets suspicious of what is happening ", writes Frazer, " he has two alternatives : he either tries to avert the attack by calling in a friendly magician or he gives in, refuses to eat and dies from mental shock believing that he is lost ". W. E. Roth, the ethnographer and physician, describes this fatal form of auto-suggestion as thanatomania, and Malinovski has seen several such cases during his stay with the Trobriand Islanders.

The primitive is equally afraid to let severed parts of his body, such as his nails or hair, or excreta, fall into the hands of his foe. He holds that whatever may happen to them would affect him in a similar way. Even the very air he breathes, his foot-prints, his shadow, or even the left-overs of his meal may be possessed of similar uncanny properties and may thus contribute to the anguish and anxieties of his daily life.

But the idea of sympathetic or telepathic magic is not confined to the operation at a distance of harmful or malignant influences. Innumerable practices of sex magic have been collected by the ethnologists in which, at least on the face of it, the sadistic-aggressive element seems to be absent.

There are charms and love potions which aim at winning the favours of a prudish belle, or of inciting the passions of a reluctant lover. A few examples quoted by Róheim may illustrate this aspect of the magic art. In Hungary the girl " lifts " the earth from the footprint of a lad and puts it down again with the toe pointing in the opposite direction. By this act she believes that she will win back her lover from another village whither he has strayed.

More in the line of telepathic magic in stricter sense, is the superstition described by Ch. S. Burne from Shropshire : " If you want to fetch a lover from a distance you must get a penny-worth of dragon's blood from the chemist and perform with it various rites. A girl who tried this fetched her husband by train from a distance. They had just had a quarrel. ' Why, whatever brought you ? ' she asked when he arrived. ' I could not rest ', he said. ' I felt as if I must come.' "

But love magic is thought to be operative without the aid of any material vehicles. We learn from Malinovski that erotic thoughts are believed to be able to act upon the mind of a distant lover though he may be hundreds of miles away, especially while he is asleep. In a collection of *Myths and Legends of the Australian Aborigines* we read of a loving couple united by " an interchange of feelings and emotions in a language that no song, no speech, or other medium can express ". A very ancient folk-tale from Western Mexico recounts how the dainty little Patayamu wandering about, fell in love with the Yellow Corn maiden. He began to think that he would elope with her. The Corn Maiden guessed his thoughts and became very alarmed. Yet she whispered to her companions : " Let us dance a little longer, I think he will soon fall asleep and then we will run away ".

Besides love and hatred reaching beyond the confines of the physical personality, the fear of death has been one of the main problems deeply stirring the imagination of primitive man. Its approach is announced by many and varied omens presaging what is about to happen to a distant friend or relation. In the ancient Egyptian tale of the *Two Brothers* the younger announced to the older one that " when the beer froze and the wine comes sour in his vessel " this would be an indication of his death. It is one of the most ancient instances of an alleged veridical communication from the dying. In the well-known tale of *The Beauty and the Beast*, Beauty learns of her far-away lover's malady in a dream and rushes to his sick bed. In a story recorded by W. Sollas among the Australian Aborigines we learn of Kaang who sent his son Cagaz to the baboon country to cut sticks for making bows. He was caught by the baboons and killed. Kaang was asleep at that time, but when he awoke he found out " by his magic " what had happened ; so he went to the baboons to revenge his son. Malinovski describes how the Trobriand Islanders believe that a fully trained Muluquasi —a witch—" by a special sense can hear, as the natives say, that a man has died at such and such a place, or that a canoe is in danger. Even a young apprenticed Yoyova will have her ' hearing ' so sharpened that she will exclaim : ' Mother, I hear a cry ! ' which means that a man is dying at some place. Or she will say ' Mother, a Waga is sinking ! ' "

A similar story is reported by Lévy-Bruhl, quoting the account of an Eskimo woman : " Mother had cooked some ribs of a walrus and was sitting eating when the bone she held suddenly began to make a noise. She was so frightened that she at once threw down the bone. I remember her face went quite white and she burst out 'something has happened to my son'. And so indeed it had. A little later they heard he was dead." Longfellow's *Hiawatha* contains the famous passage in which his hero

> Miles away among the mountains
> Heard the sudden cry of anguish,
> Heard the song of Minnehaha,
> Calling to him in the darkness,

announcing to him her death. We shall see on a later page that there is a striking similarity of these narratives with examples of alleged telepathy from the dying, reported in the literature of psychical research.

In similar accounts originating from a higher level of civilisation the primitive, magic element more and more recedes into the background, whilst the demarcation line between the natural and the supernatural becomes more easily discernible. Such happenings, real or imaginary—as we just described—assume an increasingly awe-inspiring character. Their occurrence is ascribed to the intervention of divine agencies, confined to exceptional occasions or to places of worship and sanctuaries and they are being made the exclusive concern of a privileged priestly cast—the successors of the primitive medicine men or magicians. The priest may in turn seek to gain increasing power over the forces which he claims to possess. He may try to control their operation through special devices, mental or physical, aided if necessary by deliberate fraud and trickery.

One of the methods used by the ancient Egyptian, Greek or Roman priests and necromancers was the so-called temple sleep. It was believed to impart telepathic, clairvoyant or prophetic dreams upon the sleeper, or to make him susceptible to the healing powers of the priest in charge of the shrine. In the case of the famous oracles of Delphi or Dodona the Pythonesses were exposed to narcotising vapours which were held to promote their divinatory powers. In other cases, trance was achieved by chewing different herbs or roots, or by drinking water possessed of magic powers. The ancient Mexican priests used to intoxicate the *Listeners to the Majas* with cocaine, tobacco, or pejotl, the drug that makes "the eyes enchanted", the mother substance of mescaline of modern pharmacopœia. Other devices applied were orgiastic dances performed until the dancers collapsed from final exhaustion, prolonged fasting, vigils, sexual abstinence, self-castigation and partial strangulation resulting in cerebral anaemia and loss of consciousness.

The ancient Yogis resorted to a variety of similar practices. They comprise methods which are still being widely used in modern European folk-lore, including the familiar semi-scientific methods of inducing hypnotic sleep. The Yogi keeps gazing on a definite point: on the tip of his nose or on his navel, until his eyes become tired and filled with tears, and he ultimately loses consciousness and falls into catalepsy. This state is the so-called Yoga sleep and one of the favourite methods of achieving tapas which is claimed to confer the faculties of thought reading, clairvoyance and precognition upon the devotee.

Other physical aids serving the same purpose are various bodily attitudes named *asana*, holding the breath in a state between inhalation and exhalation, counting the respirations, and the like. All this has to be tried out in strict seclusion from the outer world, in complete silence and darkness. But all these practices had to be raised to a higher level through combination with spiritual meditation. This was held to lead to complete emancipation from the senses and to open up the gates of the Unseen World.

Similar tendencies can be traced in many of the higher religions of our day when they commend the practice of spiritual meditation and absorption in prayer as a source of higher revelation leading to what is described as the mystic union with the divinity. But they, too, do not altogether dispense with the aid of various physical devices in order to promote the requisite detached state of mind. We may recall the praying wheel of the Tibetan monks, the phylactery of the Jews, the rosary of the Catholic worshipper.

The conviction that ordinary sleep is a source of divinatory powers has been a matter of self-evidence to the ancient Chinese, Egyptians, Jews and Greeks, and has remained a popular belief up to present days. There are innumerable anecdotal accounts in the classical literature bearing out this point. I need only quote the well-known legend of Calpurnia's dream on the night preceding Caesar's assassination. Tradition holds that she dreamt that the roof of the house had fallen in and that her husband, stabbed by his enemies, was dying in her arms. She saw Caesar's statue

> Whence like a fountain with a hundred spouts
> Did run pure blood and many lusty Romans
> Came running and did bathe their hands in it.
> And those does she apply for warnings and portents
> And evils imminent.

A modern counterpart of Plutarch's account and its Shakespearean transcription is contained in President Lincoln's biography by Ward Hill Laman. According to Laman, Lincoln described a premonitory dream he had a few weeks prior to his assassination as follows: "There seemed to be death-like stillness about me . . . then I heard subdued sobs, as if a number of people were weeping. I thought I left my bed and wandered downstairs. There, the silence was broken by the same pitiful sobbing but the mourners were invisible. I went from room to room; no living person was inside, but the same mournful sound of distress met me as I passed along . . . I was puzzled and alarmed. What could be the meaning of all this . . . ? I arrived at the East room which I entered. There I met a sickening surprise. Before me was a catafalque on which rested a corpse wrapped in funeral vestments. Around it were stationed soldiers who were acting as guards; and there was a throng of people, some gazing mournfully upon the corpse whose face was covered, others weeping pitifully. 'Who is dead in the White House?' the dreamer asks. 'The President . . . He was killed by an assassin.'" And Lincoln added, so concludes Ward Hill Laman's report: "I slept no more that night and was strangely annoyed by the dream ever since".

Another famous anecdote from ancient times is concerned with the divinatory powers attributed to the Delphic Oracle. The story rests with the dubious authority of Herodotus and must be regarded as largely fictitious: Croesus, King of Lydia, wished to procure the sanction of the Gods for his war on Cyrus, but before invoking the advice of the renowned oracles of his time he decided to put them to the test and accordingly despatched six envoys to six oracles, fixing a certain date on which they were to ask what Croesus, in his palace at Sardes, was doing at the particular moment. He had chosen an action which he assumed would be beyond all possible conjecture. All oracles but one failed completely. One produced what would now be described as a " near miss ". Delphi won the race. This was what it said :

> I can count the sands and I can measure the Ocean,
> I have ears for the silent, and know what the dumb man meaneth
> Lo ! On my sense there striketh the smell of a shell-covered Tortoise
> Boiling now on fire with the flesh of a lamb in a cauldron.
> Brass in the vessel below and brass the cover above it.

Herodotus recounts that Croesus, on the appointed day, at the very same time, " had set himself what was most impossible to conceive of his doing, and then, waiting until the day agreed on came, he acted as he had determined. He took a tortoise and a lamb and cutting them in pieces with his own hands boiled them both together in a brazen cauldron covered over with a lid which was also of brass. "

I emphasised that Herodotus' narrative can certainly not be regarded as documentary evidence of an historic event, but it reflects a new attitude towards the problem of alleged supernormal phenomena : the attitude of the scientifically minded investigator, who takes nothing for granted unless he puts it to an empirical test. The question whether the story of Croesus and the Delphic oracle does, or does not, contain a grain of truth is immaterial ; the point is that it constitutes the first connecting link between the primitive notion of telepathic magic and the modern rational approach to the problem of paranormal cognition.

What, then, is the correlation between the primitive concept of telepathic or sympathetic magic and its modern counterpart, telepathy in stricter sense, and what is the difference between them ? Clearly, the primitive concept covers a much wider range of phenomena. It refers to events, mental or physical, whose action at a distance is asserted. It comprises the belief in the telepathic implications of actions, of symbolic gestures such as rites and ceremonies or of spoken words such as spells and incantations, as well as of unformulated thoughts or ideas. By contrast, the concept of telepathy in the modern sense suggests nothing else than the telepathic activity of thoughts and other mental processes.

A further point of difference refers to the subject-matter of telepathic " transmission ". We intimated that the mainspring of telepathic and sympathetic magic has been man's desire to control the forces of nature and the minds of his fellow-men. It revolves around the poles of fear and self-assertion, of hatred and love. Telepathic magic is charged with the deepest passions that stirred the lives of primitive men ; indeed, it is the vehicle by which he seeks to give vent to his pent-up emotions, by which he believes he is able to impose his will upon the world around him. Another significant point was brought out by Róheim, who upon examining primitive mentality from the psychoanalytical point of view, emphasised the prevailing sadistic-agressive character of the magic art and showed that this is largely due to primitive man's own repressed sadistic-aggressive tendencies and their projection on to his fellow-men. Telepathic magic, whatever its nature, has in this way a marked emotional emphasis. It is the expression of man's passionate desire to reach out beyond the limited range of his physical personality and to impose his will upon the world around him.

By contrast, there is nothing left in the modern notion of telepathy of this primitive, sadistic-aggressive element. If it ever contained such an ingredient, it has been thoroughly purged of its presence. Indeed, telepathy in the modern sense has either been reduced to a harmless social game, to a feature of an engaging vaudeville production, or, in its latest disguise as Professor Rhine's extra-sensory perception, to the subject of fascinating scientific inquiry, conducted with all the ingenuity of the modern laboratory approach. In any case, it has become a thoroughly civilised affair, stripped of most of its emotional colouring and barely recognisable as a descendant of its forerunner in bygone times.

But whilst modern psychical research has been at great pains to remove the last vestiges of the ancient magic and animistic belief from its subject-matter and to raise the preoccupation with it to the standard of a recognised branch of science, there has remained a redoubtable compartment on the outer fringes as it were of contemporary civilisation in which a substantial part of primitive mentality seems to have survived. It is occupied by the sect of the spiritualists. It is true that spiritualistic doctrine, too, has tried hard to conceal its doubtful parentage and to make concessions to the temper of modern times. It adopted a high sounding semi-scientific nomenclature, it borrowed some of the concepts of nineteenth-century romanticism and philosophy, but in so doing it only changed its garment and otherwise maintained most of the original tenets of the ancient primitive creed. It still believes in personal survival after death, in the possibility of mind acting directly upon matter and, above all, of thought and action at a distance. In the spiritualist seance room what was once proclaimed as demoniacal possession is still being produced to order ; prophecy and divination is being proffered in a new disguise to credulous clients ; tables are tilted, articles hurled through the air, musical instruments sounded by invisible forces, physical shapes emerge from the dark leaving palpable imprints in plaster of paris moulds, and a mysterious soul-substance is being secreted from the medium's mouth or other bodily openings.

It is true that, so far, none of these so-called physical phenomena has stood the test of closer examination. Levitation of objects turned out to be manipulated by fraudulent tricks, spirit photographs revealed as spurious and the ectoplasma produced by the entranced medium was found to consist of scraps of mousseline tissue. However, all the evidence afforded against the genuineness of the phenomena, all the mediums exposed for fraud and deception have not been able to shake the faith of the modern primitives. The spiritualist remains inaccessible to arguments wherever his deeply rooted beliefs and pre-conceived ideas are concerned. In the midst of twentieth-century civilisation he lives on an island on which for all practical intents and purposes the psychological flora and fauna of a past age has survived. Edward Tylor, one of the first explorers of this submerged Atlantis of the Soul, pointed out as long as sixty years ago that animism and magic have in fact never ceased to be latent propensities in the minds of civilised peoples. He describes spiritualism " as a direct revival from regions of savage philosophy and peasant folklore ". It revives practices which have roots deep in the very stratum of the world outlook of prehistoric man. Thus, it comes about that in the spiritualistic seance room " the world is again swarming with intelligent and powerful disembodied spiritual beings whose direct action on thought and matter is confidently asserted ".

There can be little wonder, then, that all the claims regarding so-called supernormal phenomena put forward by the pioneers of psychical research in the eighties of the past century met with profound scepticism on the part of both scientists and the general public. Most observations of alleged telepathy, clairvoyance, veridical dreams, etc., seemed to bear the stigmata of crude superstitions and unfounded beliefs, exposed by the new rational approach to science and philosophy. The doubtful extraction of the claimed phenomena was itself an ambiguous recommendation and their close correlation with the ridiculous mumbo-jumbo of the spiritualistic seance room additional reason for distrust. To this came what was described as the " intrinsic improbability " of the observations, their flagrant contradiction to the established laws of nature, to the familiar body of our experience, in a word to common sense. Indeed, to the rationalistic trend of nineteenth-century science and philosophy the slightest doubt in the infallibility of its basic concepts appeared worse than heresy and was punished with the worst punishment that could be meted out to a man of science or letters : with ridicule. James Frazer and Edward Tylor, the pioneers of anthropology of the past century, stressed the correspondence of the doctrines proclaimed by Frederic Myers and his associates with the " monstrous farrago " of the magic and animistic creed. " Whatever doubts science may entertain as to the possibility of action at a distance, magic has none ; faith in telepathy is one of its first principles. A modern advocate of supernormal phenomena would have no difficulty in persuading a savage," writes Frazer in his *Golden Bough*.

All the greater were the difficulties of F. Myers and his associates in trying to persuade Frazer and his contemporaries. No lesser an authority than the German physicist Helmholtz emphatically declared : " Neither the testimony of all the Fellows of the Royal Society, nor even the evidence of my own senses could lead me to believe in the transmission of thoughts from one person to another independently of the recognised channels of sensation ". He was seconded by Lord Kelvin in this country who dismissed all such reports as being due to " bad observation chiefly, mixed up with the effects of wilful imposture ". Henry Maudsley, in his book entitled *Natural Causes and Supernatural Seeming*, wrote in a similar vein. And even as recently as 1939 Wilhelm Weygandt, the German psychiatrist, assumed the same uncompromising attitude.

Other investigators were ready to compromise. They accepted the evidence in favour of such unusual occurrences as thought-reading or thought-transference, but ascribed it largely to a hyperesthesia of the senses, to the appreciation of " subliminal " sensory clues, such as unconscious whispering, or to an uncanny ability of muscle-reading. Explanations like these took at least the sting of the irrational out of the phenomena. They facilitated their classification alongside such other curiosities of man's psychic life as optical illusions, hallucinations, hyperfunctions of the dream, etc. The rest could conveniently be explained as faulty observation or deliberate deception.

But the decisive blow against the feasibility of alleged supernormal phenomena was delivered by the psychoanalytic doctrine. I have already hinted that in the view of Freud and his disciples belief in telepathy, clairvoyance, etc., is nothing but a feature of primitive mentality, common to the savage, the child and the neurotic patient. This belief is largely due to an over-estimation of our mental processes. Primitive man finds that his thoughts reflect in some way the order of things in the outer world and he jumps to the conclusion that he is therefore able to control and dominate them with his will. This is the fallacy of what Freud described as *omnipotence of thought*. In his *Totem and Tabu* he gives a brilliant exposition of this theory applied to various aspects of animism and magic, and their reflection in certain tribal customs of primitive man, in the day-dreams and phantasies of the child, and in the clinical picture of the obsessional neurosis. Freud mentions a patient of this type who confessed to him that " whenever he uttered a half-meant imprecation against a stranger he could expect him to die soon thereafter and burden him with the responsibility of his death ".

Since Freud first called attention to observations of this kind, a great deal of evidence has been adduced confirming the striking similarity between primitive mentality and the thinking of neurotic patients of the obsessional-compulsory type. This similarity is indeed so remarkable that it is apt to show the whole problem of alleged supernormal phenomena in a new light and to confirm the suspicion that it is not so much the problem of telepathy or paranormal cognition, or whatever it be termed, that calls for closer investigation, as the very sanity of those asserting its existence. In fact, the psychoanalysis of neurotic patients, as well as of certain psychotics, invariably reveals the presence of a craving for Freud's "omnipotence of thought", for "omniscience". H. Hitschman, one of Freud's early associates, in a study devoted to our problem, is satisfied that belief in telepathy is itself nothing else than a psychological symptom, a manifestation of man's narcissistic libido organisation, of his wishful thinking based on the pleasure principle.

This is, in a nutshell, the psychoanalytic interpretation of primitive mentality, and there can be little doubt that it is in good keeping with the general trend of contemporary medical psychology. It fits the case not only of the ancient magic and animistic creed, but also most of the familiar facts of normal and abnormal psychology. There is only one flaw in the psychoanalytic reasoning. A small band of amateur investigators and professional scientists, unperturbed by the arguments which have been put forward against the possibility of telepathy and related phenomena, have furnished incontrovertible evidence which proves their existence.

Chapter II

WHAT ARE THE FACTS?

WHAT then, are the facts?

The answer to this question has been the quest of more than sixty years of psychical research inaugurated by a few amateur investigators whose work was in turn furthered and co-ordinated by various scientific societies. More recently, psychical research, or parapsychology, has reached the stage of academic respectability: it is being sponsored and subsidised by universities both in the United States of America, and in this country, while half a dozen journals report regularly on the advances of the new science and the results of a wide variety of investigations carried out by research workers specially trained in statistical methods and experimental psychology are gaining increasing publicity among scientists and the general public.

I do not propose to attempt anything like a complete survey of this work in the present book: its history has already been recorded by such authorities as C. Richet in France, and G. N. M. Tyrrell and Professor H. H. Price in this country. Several standard works edited by J. B. Rhine and his co-workers in the United States give an excellent survey of the whole field covered during the past decades. For the present purpose, therefore, it will suffice to select a few representative examples of the phenomena ranging from the first anecdotal accounts by the early workers, of more or less authenticated experiments of what may be called the pre-scientific period, up to the well-established and statistically evaluated modern laboratory experiments of psychical research.

It must be admitted that the evidential value of this material is unequal. Indeed, it has become customary among mathematically minded investigators to exclude altogether accounts of the first type from a serious inquiry and to rely exclusively on the evidence of quantitative laboratory experiments. Later, we shall discuss how far this attitude is justifiable, but just now it will be as well to begin by discussing a few typical examples of so-called spontaneous phenomena such as can be observed in everyday life.

Alleged telepathy from the dying is a typical instance of this kind. One of the classics of the literature of psychical research, *The Phantasms of the Living*, by Myers, Gurney and Podmore, contains scores of accounts of this type. The story usually reads as follows :—

Mr. X., suddenly awaking from sleep, hears a voice crying for help, it may be calling his name or merely sighing in a barely perceptible manner. He is immediately aware that an absent friend, or relation, is in a state of crisis, in mortal danger, or has met with an accident. In some cases this experience is in the nature of an apparition, that is, of a visual hallucination in which the picture of a certain person appears before his mind's eye as if endeavouring to speak, or to convey by its expression the idea of impending peril, illness or death. Sometimes the scene is described in great detail and contains information which can be verified on subsequent inquiry. In other cases it is merely a spasm of sudden, baseless anxiety, apparently connected with an indefinite danger threatening the absent friend, and although detailed information may be lacking, subsequent inquiry may show that the apprehension raised by the "premonition" was justified.

There are many obvious objections to a telepathic interpretation of such experiences. For instance, it can be argued that the evidence is unsatisfactory; that the testimony of casual and unqualified witnesses fails to possess scientific validity, or that accounts by persons who have themselves passed through a state of worry or anxiety are unreliable. Moreover, it is widely recognised that faulty recollections, misrepresentation of trivial occurrences after the event are a common source of error in all walks of life and particularly so in psychical research. Furthermore, it has rightly been stated that "positive" cases are more likely to be specially noted, whilst "negative" ones pass unnoticed and consequently fail to counterbalance the false impression created by a few spectacular chance happenings.

It can be also argued that accounts of spontaneous occurrences of all kinds, including alleged telepathy from the dying, bear a suspicious resemblance to such primitive beliefs and superstitions as were discussed in the previous chapter. I may recall the ancient Egyptian story of the *Two Brothers;* the fairy tale of *The Beauty and the Beast;* Malinovsky's report of the *Yoyova* who can hear the death-yell of a man drowning in a river miles away. All these narratives are wont to be dismissed as figments of imagination characteristic of primitive mentality.

On the other hand, we have to note that there is an increasing number of instances in the literature of what are claimed to be true telepathic, or otherwise "supernormal" occurrences in primitive peoples. I need only mention that much discussed case of the Australian Bush telegraph; the remarkable exploits of Indian Yogis and Tibetan monks. It is true that all these reports are still more difficult to verify than similar observations made under civilised conditions. Indeed, whenever we try to assess the part played by telepathy in trivial occurrences in our daily life we are up against the difficulty of mere fact-finding. There is the case of letters posted precisely at the same time by far distant friends under circumstances which seem to exclude chance coincidence or a common "inducing" factor. There are reports of a person turning round when he is looked at from behind or of cases in which when a long forgotten friend turns up round the street corner at precisely the moment you happened to think of him, or her, as the case may be. The *Proceedings of the Society for Psychical Research* contain hundreds of observations of apparent telepathy of this kind.

A great many unsuccessful attempts have been made to put these observations to the test. There is, however, a series of earlier experiments closely approximating to the conditions of everyday life which are deserving of mention. They were carried out by Professor Gilbert Murray and members of his family, and largely followed the pattern of the then popular "guessing game". Reports of these experiments were published in detail by Mrs. H. Sidgwick in the *Proceedings of the Society for Psychical Research.* The procedure was as follows:—

Professor Murray would leave the family circle which had gathered in the drawing-room, and proceed into another room out of earshot. The rest of the family agreed on thinking of some past incident, dramatic or trivial, connected with one of those present, or with an absent friend. Alternatively, a passage from a book, or a purely imaginary event was selected.

Professor Murray would then be called back into the room and asked to guess of what the others were thinking.

Reasonable precautions were taken to rule out sensory clues or information gained through other normal channels, and in view of the unquestionable *bona fides* of the participants collusion could be safely ruled out. Further, the wide, indeed infinite, variety of items from among which both the agents and the percipient were at liberty to choose, made the accounting for correct guesses by chance coincidence highly improbable. In addition, careful records of the experiments were taken by a reliable shorthand-typist. An example may illustrate the procedure :

Mrs. Arnold Toynbee—Professor Murray's daughter—is the agent : she thinks of the beginning of a story by Dostojevsky in which the dog of a poor old man is dying in a restaurant.

Professor Murray : "I think it's a thing in a book. A very miserable old man, I think, is doing something with a dead dog. A very unhappy one. I rather think it's a restaurant and people are mocking, and then they are sorry and want to be kind. Of the nationality I am not sure. I have a feeling it is a sort of Gorki thing. I have a feeling it is something Russian."

Experiments of this kind were conducted over a period of years with varying results. In some of them the percipient's guesses were even more convincing than in the above example. For instance, when he correctly reproduced the first line of a poem selected by the agent, or when he, in great detail, described a particularly comical incident which occurred to a member of his family.

In other cases his guess was much less accurate, and Professor Murray seemed able to catch little more than the general atmosphere, or an insignificant detail, from a complex situation. Such "near misses" are certainly less convincing than a fully correct guess, but we shall see on a later page that they are of even greater psychological interest.

On one occasion Mr. Patrick Murray thought of the lion in the zoo trying to reach a large piece of meat just outside the cage.

Professor Murray: "A sort of smell of wild animals. Something grabbing through the bars at a piece of meat at a zoo. Don't know the animal."

Again, in other cases he seemed to miss the point completely. The agent had thought of an operating room in which he was being operated on.

Professor Murray: "I got an impression of a theatre. No. I can't get it. I am now guessing. . . ."

It will be noticed, however, that there exists an unmistakable correspondence between operation room and operation theatre, although the connection is admittedly too loose to permit any definite conclusions.

The peculiar vague correlation between the agent's "target" idea and the percipient's guess, has been one of the principal difficulties of such early experiments in telepathy as were first described in 1886 by Myers, Gurney and Podmore in their *Phantasms of the Living*. It has remained the chief stumbling block in numerous attempts at improving upon the technique of experiments with so-called freely chosen material.

The French chemical engineer René Warcollier devoted twenty-five years of laborious research to this task. He claims the best results in group experiments with telepathic drawings. Two examples may illustrate his technique:

One of his collaborators, playing the part of an agent, looked at a print which represented the Iron Serpent of Duesseldorf, a queer, surrealistic monument erected on the quay of a river. Madame S., acting as percipient, received first the impression of a serpent, "of something that 'writhes' and then goes noisily up and away, perhaps an airplane".

Her own drawing clearly conveys the picture of a serpent.

On another occasion Warcollier himself was the agent, and he looked at the picture of a hangar with an airship in it. In a sketch reproducing his own impression he drew a rough outline of the airship only. Madame S., the percipient, again seems to miss the real thing. She sketches a wall with ladders placed alongside it, adding a plumb-line to her drawing to express symbolically the inclination of the ladder. At first sight her drawing seems to bear no resemblance to the original. Yet, on analysis, it is clear—at least in the view of Warcollier—that here, again, the telepathic copy actually reproduces the lateral supports of the hangar which may then easily be mistaken for ladders leaning against a wall.

From observations like these Warcollier draws a number of interesting conclusions. He suggests that it is precisely what the agent does not think of transmitting which is most successfully transmitted : parts instead of the whole, elements which remain unnoticed and which may then appear distorted in such a manner as to make them barely recognisable. Yet, as in the case of Professor Murray's experiments, the wide scope given to subjective interpretation is evident.

In some of the tests reproduced in Warcollier's book the close correspondence between the original and the telepathic copy is undeniable ; in others it is more than questionable. Warcollier fails to offer a reliable standard of assessment, and in this respect his material is hardly more convincing than that of his predecessors.

The same objection applies to more recent investigators working along similar lines. Upton Sinclair's book on *Mental Radio* is a case in point. But although most of his experiments were carried out under still less stringent conditions than the Warcollier tests, here, too, the *bona fides* of the experimenters is beyond doubt, and some of the observations described are highly suggestive of telepathy.

In one of the experiments described it was arranged that Mrs. Sinclair and her brother should make drawings on paper at an appointed time whilst they were staying in different towns miles apart. Sinclair reproduces a number of drawings thus obtained, some of them showing a striking correspondence. In one instance, both subjects drew a chair, in another identical table forks. But in the Sinclair series, too, there is a tendency for the percipient's guess to slip from the essential to the accidental, and a sceptic may well regard the author's interpretations equivocal and the similarities claimed unconvincing. Moreover, it goes without saying that here, again, the objection of chance coincidence cannot lightly be dismissed.

A further shortcoming of all experiments of this kind is their persistent failure to materialise " to command ". They cannot be repeated at will, and it has rightly been argued that the better the experimental conditions, the stricter the safeguards against fraud, errors of observation or self-deception, the more elusive are the results obtained. On the other hand, it has often been noted that the slacker the precautionary measures taken, the poorer the obtaining experimental conditions, the more spectacular is the subject performance.

There is another flaw, less commonly realised, which seems to be inherent in the usual experiments with telepathy. The telepathy hypothesis assumes that under favourable conditions, thoughts, ideas or other mental contents are being perceived by a percipient without the aid of the recognised sensory channels. In the examples so far reviewed the experimenter's attention was focussed on a deliberately selected set of items, and if he were able to identify a similar set of items in another person's mental content, he was satisfied that telepathy had taken place.

But, on what grounds does he arrive at this conclusion? When is he safe in assuming that he has been focussing his attention on the right things? Is he altogether justified in taking it for granted that his percipient is able (or willing) to obey the rules of the game which he is expected to play and to concentrate upon the items which he is supposed to reproduce in a telepathic way? How can the experimenter preclude the possibility that his subject might tap the agent's mental content at a different level, as it were, or worse still, that the percipient might be side-tracked upon some mental content of his own, instead of that of the agent?

Again, experiments with what is called freely chosen material are based on the presupposition that the agent is at liberty to choose whatever item he intends to concentrate upon, and to shut out any other item from his mind. However, this assumption is totally arbitrary. There is nothing to prevent thoughts, ideas or expectations, not immediately concerned with the proposed test, from entering the agent's mind. It may even so happen that an item from the mind of a person other than the selected agent may affect the mind of the percipient and thus gate-crash into the experimental situation. Indeed, it is clear that telepathic leakage of this kind can hardly be prevented whatever its source, and that its role is difficult to assess in any given experiment.

However, on reading the records of the early workers in telepathy it is obvious that most of them have failed to make proper allowance for the occurrence of telepathic leakage, although it is obvious that, from the very nature of the telepathy hypothesis, such a possibility should have been taken into account.

There can be no doubt that telepathic leakage originating from unconscious wishes or expectations of either the experimenter or of any other person concerned with the tests may easily modify their outcome and even determine results in a decisive way. We shall refer to such influences from outside the pre-arranged experimental situation under the heading of para-experimental telepathy and we shall see that this factor may indeed be an important source of error not only in the assessment of paranormal cognition, but also of the results of psychological observations in general.

However, the principal objection which can be raised to experiments in telepathy with freely chosen material is the objection of chance coincidence. It has rightly been argued that positive observations, however striking they appear, fail to carry conviction so long as there is no way to determine the probability, or improbability, of an actual "hit" by the statistical method. The early workers were well aware of this difficulty, but relying as they were on results derived from freely chosen material, they were unable to develop a method of mathematical evaluation. An important step in this direction was made by Miss Ina Jephson, a member of the Society for Psychical Research as far back as 1928. In association with Professor R. A. Fisher she worked out a method of card calling tests which readily lent themselves to statistical assessment. Experiments of this type eliminate most of the ambiguity of the earlier tests. The percipient's guess is either right or wrong. There is no third alternative, no scope for subjective interpretation, and accordingly the chances of failure or success can be expressed in unequivocal mathematical terms.

The credit of having raised this technique to the standard of an unassailable scientific method undoubtedly goes to Dr. J. B. Rhine of Duke University, Durham, N.C., and there is a wide consensus of opinion that his work marks the beginning of a new era of parapsychology. Rhine used for his experiments a pack of twenty-five cards, containing five sets of five different symbols : a star, a cross, wavy lines, a circle and a square.

Special precautions were taken by the makers of these so-called Zener cards to rule out distinguishing marks on their backs which might give the game away. In addition, in certain tests various mechanical shuffling devices were used to prevent errors due to faulty shuffling of the packs.

According to the laws of probability calculation the odds for rightly guessing such a card symbol are one in five. More than five correct guesses in a series of twenty-five cards are in excess of mere chance expectation. Guided by this principle Rhine was able to assess the deviation of scores from chance and to express results obtained in such well defined terms as the standard deviation, the critical ratio, etc.

The method of evaluation has since developed into a science of its own, and the reader wishing to obtain further information may be referred to the relevant literature. The point is, that the statistical approach has, as a matter of fact, furnished a reliable standard for determining the extra-chance nature of scores.

In pursuance of this work, Rhine and his co-workers devised a number of safeguards to secure water-tight experimental conditions, to exclude sensory clues, deception or self-deception, or errors of recording. Among the measures taken I may only mention : new packs of cards were used for each series of experiments ; the packs were supplied in sealed envelopes, opaque screens separated agent from percipient when seated in the same room, the scores were recorded in ink by two independent witnesses, the operator being constantly present during the whole testing period.

In a series of experiments carried out along these lines by Pratt and Woodruff, stamped and consecutively numbered record sheets were used. Locked boxes were prepared to receive the record sheets immediately after they were completed. Furthermore, a third observer was called upon to check the records before they were deposited in the locked box. The assessment was done by " independent counting of hits, direct from the cards, and complete record scores, independently retained by each experimenter ".

Pratt and Woodruff report that " under these elaborate

conditions 60,000 trials were made and gave a positive deviation of 489 and a critical ratio of 4·99 ". That is to say, the total number of guesses in excess of chance expectation was 489, or a figure enormously greater than is expected from chance alone. The odds against such happenings can be expressed in astronomical figures only.

Rhine and his co-workers conclude from the results of many hundreds of thousands of tests carried out by a number of experimenters under varied conditions, (1) " that they are extra-chance in nature ; (2) that the research has adduced large blocks of extra-chance data under conditions which, according to the procedure described, appeared to have excluded sensory clues to the satisfaction of all requirements ; (3) that in several instances in which the research crucially excluded explanation by chance or by sensory clues, the conditions were such as to prohibit clerical errors from affecting the deviation ". Rhine feels justified, therefore, in regarding the results summarised in his report as incontrovertible evidence of what he termed extra-sensory perception.

But the statistical method has more than merely established the fact of paranormal cognition. By varying the experimental arrangements Rhine could show that many of his subjects could guess the target card even though it was not being looked at by an agent. This he described as E.S.P. under clairvoyant conditions. Rhine and his co-workers were able to separate this form of extra-sensory perception from experiments under conditions of so-called pure telepathy. In these latter experiments the percipient has to guess not at a real card picked out of the pack, but at the mental picture of a card symbol which the agent was thinking of. Written records of the agent's choice of a card symbol were made only after the percipient had registered his guess. The experimenter was thus able to distinguish between paranormal cognition of clairvoyant and telepathic type, by contrast to the early workers in psychical research whose experiments were largely amenable to two alternative interpretations.

But the final appreciation of Rhine's results was open to an objection which he was the first to raise. E.S.P. under clairvoyant conditions implies direct knowledge or direct awareness of things in the outer world, without the aid of the ordinary sensory channels and without reference to the mental contents of another person. Yet, on merely logical grounds it might well be argued that the percipient may just as well be able to anticipate in some unaccountable way the purely mental event of the subsequent check-up by the experimenter of the percipient's score. This is certainly nothing but a hypothetical conjecture but difficult to disprove. In any case, experiments conducted by Rhine and his co-workers regarding the existence of precognitive abilities were difficult to interpret.

However, two series of experiments carried out in this country, apparently furnished the missing link in Rhine's chain of reasoning. The story begins with a series of drawing tests conducted by Whately Carington in Cambridge. They were originally devised along the lines of the older drawing tests but with a greatly improved technique. Carington's procedure was as follows: He put up a drawing in his study made by himself, or his wife, just before the experiment. The drawing was left there overnight, the possibility being strictly ruled out that it could be seen by any other person. The subject of the drawing was chosen by a random method from a dictionary, the relevant page of which was suggested by selecting a number from logarithmic tables, again in a random way. About two hundred and fifty percipients in various localities in and outside this country were instructed to make attempts at reproducing the picture wherever they happened to be on the same night. This procedure was repeated for ten successive nights with ten different drawings selected in a similar way and displayed under conditions of strictest privacy.

In January, 1944, Whately Carington published in America a catalogue of thousands of drawings made by his subjects in order to find out in a statistically assessable manner what sort of drawings they would produce outside the experimental situation. By means of this catalogue he was able to determine the probability of each drawing produced by a percipient being due to chance alone. In earlier experiments the drawings made by his percipients under telepathic conditions were sent to an umpire who marked their degree of similarity, or otherwise, with the originals. All details of the method of marking, assessment, etc., cannot be described here. They must be gathered from Carington's original publication. Be it sufficient to remark that his experiments seem indeed to represent a decisive step towards a method of repeatable and statistically assessable E.S.P. tests far superior to all earlier experiments with telepathic drawings.

The matching of the drawings by the umpire at the end of the ten days confronted Carington with a surprise. A high degree of similarity between a certain proportion of originals and their presumed reproductions was found, far exceeding anything like chance expectation. Yet a qualification had to be made.

The method of matching was based on the telepathy hypothesis; that is, on the assumption that "if a percipient as a result of paranormal cognitive processes obtains a correct impression of an original which he cannot see, he will do so (or at least is most likely to do so) on the same occasion on which the said original is displayed". The matching of the drawings revealed, however, that this assumption was not true. In fact, there was a large number of "reproductions" which seemed to match originals drawn and displayed on another night, that is, *before* or *after* the respective percipients attempted their reproduction and, of course, after or before, the agents were concerned with "sending" the relevant images, or even at a time when a selection by the random method had not yet taken place. In other words, the correct guess did not necessarily coincide temporally with the display of the drawing supposed to be reproduced in a telepathic way.

For instance, Mr. Carington on Tuesday evening drew a buffalo, as suggested by the random consultation of the dictionary, yet, Mr. X., the percipient in North Carolina, had already "reproduced" such a picture on Monday! It will be noted that on Monday Mr. Carington could by no means foresee what would be the picture he was going to draw on Tuesday. In this way "ordinary" telepathy could not account for the results achieved. The correct guesses had to be ascribed to some unexpected faculty of pre-cognition, as Carington put it, or to a faculty of retro-cognition, if the reproduction was found to match the original displayed the previous night.

We must accept these findings, bewildering though they be,

as facts vouched for by scientists of such standing as Dr. C. D. Broad, Dr. R. H. Thouless and Professor H. H. Price, who were partly responsible for the assessments of the results. They were further corroborated by a series of card-calling tests carried out by S. G. Soal and K. M. Goldney in London.

Soal's earlier experiments had the limited objective of duplicating Professor Rhine's card-calling tests, and results at first were disappointing. None of his percipients appeared to show evidence of E.S.P., but on re-examining his records for the possibility of pre-cognitve hits, as suggested by Carington, he met with a surprise ; the revision showed that with two of his 160 subjects there was definite evidence of pre-cognitive and—as it were—post-cognitive guesses. These findings prompted Soal to resume experiments with one of his successful subjects, Mr. B. S., under rigorous experimental conditions. They corroborated the results of the earlier series. Mr. B. S., tested under conditions of pure telepathy, showed indeed a tendency to score hits far in excess of chance expectation—not on the card which was looked at by the agent " now "—but on the card which was the *next* to be selected by a random method, and of which the agent could have no conceivable knowledge at the time the percipient was registering his guess. Mr. B. S.'s pre-cognitive span amounted to between two and three and a half seconds, accumulating over two and a half years experiments to odds against chance of 10^{35} to 1. In other series his scores had a bias towards post-cognitive guesses, although the deviation in this direction was much less sustained.

A tentative interpretation of these unexpected findings will follow on a later page. Here it will be sufficient to remark that, taken as a whole, the evidence amassed undoubtedly confirms the claim of Dr. Rhine and his associates that extra-sensory perception must be regarded as an established fact, or that " the reality of the phenomena is proved as certainly as anything in psychical research is proved ", as Dr. Thouless put it in a recent Presidential Address to the Society for Psychical Research.

A further important fact revealed by the experiments with the Zener cards, telepathic drawings, etc., is that the results are independent of the materials used. Rhine worked with geometrical symbols printed on cards; Soal and Goldney used coloured pictures of five animals; others chose letters of the alphabet, lotto numbers, or the like. G. N. M. Tyrrell evolved an ingenious mechanical device which may be described here in brief. It consists of five small boxes into which the agent at random inserts the end of a pointer. The percipient, sitting behind a screen, tries to guess the box to which the experimenter is pointing. The apparatus, in its latest version, works in combination with an electrical selector device which rules out a possible tendency on the part of the experimenter to give way to preference habits in pointing to particular boxes which would yield "combinatory clues" to the percipient. Tyrrell's results have been subjected to criticism regarding the statistical assessment of scores. In this respect I do not feel competent to pass judgment. The fact remains, that one of his subjects, Miss G. J., was able to score far in excess of chance expectation. In 30,000 trials she achieved 30 per cent. of correct guesses, as against a chance probability of 20 per cent. Mr. Tyrrell's results are in this way an interesting counterpart of Rhine's experiments and at the same time corroborative evidence of his findings.

Another point upon which light is thrown by the method of mass experiments is the factor of distance and intervening screens or other obstacles. The experiments were carried out with agent and percipient seated in the same room, but separated by curtains, or by opaque screens made of a variety of materials. They were repeated with the same subjects seated in separate rooms, or buildings. The results were identical. Some of the tests at yet longer distances were less successful, but it appears that this was largely due to accidental psychological factors. To this we may add that a number of experiments with non-quantitative material succeeded at very great distances. In the Sinclair tests good results were achieved with agent and percipient thirty miles apart. Warcollier claimed results in transatlantic tests, whilst the distance in some of Carington's experiments amounted to hundreds of miles. Likewise, the majority of well-authenticated spontaneous occurrences suggest that distance and intervening materials, whatever their nature, are entirely irrelevant to the functioning of telepathy.

Another significant feature which emerges from the mass experiments is the fact that results are essentially the same whether they are carried out under pure telepathic or pure clairvoyant conditions. They are in this way both in flagrant contradiction to the familiar laws of radiation and consequently to whatever physical hypothesis may be put forward for their explanation. The close relationship between the two principal forms of extra-sensory perception is further substantiated by the observation that, with few exceptions, the identical subjects are found to be successful with both pure telepathy and clairvoyance. This goes so far that some of Rhine's percipients scored very nearly on the same extra chance level under the two alternative conditions, that their scores revealed roughly identical "distribution patterns", and that those percipients whose performance tended to decline under certain unfavourable conditions displayed this tendency in all forms of E.S.P.

These observations open up a further interesting aspect of paranormal cognition. Rhine and his co-workers tried to amplify their results by throwing light upon the psychological and physiological conditions responsible for the operation of the alleged E.S.P. faculty. They found that like any other sensory function, it is apt to decline by fatigue, boredom, by accidental indisposition or lack of spontaneous interest on the part of the subject.

Rhine also tested the reaction of individual subjects to various drugs; he states that sedatives such as sodium amytal markedly reduce the number of hits, whereas stimulants like caffein and benzedrine cancel out this effect and generally work in the opposite direction. Moreover, his observation regarding the effects of various drugs was confirmed by experiments of R. H. Thouless in this country.

Rhine concludes from these observations that both psychologically and physiologically speaking the E.S.P. faculty is closely related to ordinary sensory functions, that it is a faculty subject to definite "volitional control" and amenable to cultivation which can be improved through deliberate concentration and spoiled by external disturbing factors.

A number of objections has been put forward to these conclusions. It has been argued that the volitional nature of

E.S.P. is hardly consistent with the peculiar erratic distribution pattern of correct guesses over a large number of trials. Rhine himself has emphasised that none of his subjects is able to guess each card in each pack at will. Even with his best percipients spells of correct scoring were intermittent. For all practical intents and purposes they were, in fact, utterly unpredictable and capricious. Rhine adds that " light humours and moods " seemed to be the best for work at E.S.P., but it is clear that these can hardly be promoted by conscious concentration or deliberate effort. All this goes far to show that E.S.P. cannot be compared with normal sensory functions in point of reliability. This precisely is the reason why Rhine had to resort to the statistical method in order to demonstrate its very existence. Ordinary sensory functions, as compared with psi-phenomena have a comparatively slight margin of error. What has been described as their biological survival value is therefore incomparably higher. It may well be questioned after all, whether it is permissible to ascribe to E.S.P. any teleological significance at all at the present level of evolution, and Rhine's claim that E.S.P. can be made to work to order is obviously in need of qualification.

Summing up, it can be stated that the method of mass experiments and their statistical evaluation has proved beyond doubt the existence of paranormal cognition. It demonstrated its independence of distance, of intervening obstacles and of the materials used. It has also shown that so-called pure telepathy and pure clairvoyance can be separated from one another, although they are otherwise subject to identical psychological and physiological laws. Furthermore, it revealed that on the strength of the same evidence pre-cognitive and post-cognitive telepathy must be accepted as an established fact, however alien this may be to our familiar way of thinking.

It cannot be the task of the present inquiry to enter into a discussion of the significance of these revolutionary findings to contemporary psychology and philosophy. The time for their critical appreciation has not yet come, and however vast the mass of evidence adduced by the modern quantitative approach may be, we have to realise that it is still fragmentary, particularly in view of the fact that the laboratory method throws light only on one side of the picture, namely, on the aspect of experimental phenomena and gives no information about the causes and conditioning factors of spontaneous occurrences.

It will also be noted that even in the limited field of experimental phenomena this method fails to account for the peculiar distribution pattern of failure and success in a given series, and still less so for the causes and conditioning factors of failure or success in an individual test. Clearly, there is a gap in our understanding of the psychological background of the phenomena, spontaneous and experimental, which can only be filled by closer investigation of such well-attested spontaneous observations as come to our notice under conditions of everyday life.

Chapter III

HOW DOES IT WORK?

A FEW observations by Freud may serve as a convenient point of departure of our argument. Freud's original attitude towards alleged occult phenomena was one of guarded scepticism. I hinted in the introductory chapter at some of the reasons for this attitude. Psychoanalysis relegates the claim of telepathy into the realm of phantasy, of wishful thinking governed by the pleasure-principle, by the craving for what Freud calls omnipotence of thoughts, common to children, neurotics and primitive men. But in his *New Introductory Lectures on Psychoanalysis*, published in 1932, he describes a number of cases in which he seriously considers a telepathic interpretation.

His first observation refers to a lady of forty-three who was suffering from an unspecified neurosis. Her analysis revealed that one of the mainsprings of her illness was her fixation on her father. It was this fixation which prevented her finding happiness in her marriage. She was longing for children, but when she learned that she had to give up the hope of having any owing to an incapacitating disease of her husband, she became still more deeply entangled in her neurosis. She was twenty-seven years of age when she consulted a fortune-teller in Paris. The fortune-teller thought she was unmarried and "prophesied" that she would have two children at the age of thirty-two. But the fact is that by the time of her treatment by Professor Freud she was forty-three and had remained childless. The prophecy had in this way proved manifestly wrong. However, her analysis revealed a striking fact. It showed that there was, nevertheless, an obvious correspondence to reality in the fortune-teller's statement. The patient's mother was just thirty-two years old when, within the shortest possible interval, she gave birth to two children during the same year, after having almost given up hope of bearing children at her age.

From the psychoanalytical point of view it was clear that

the patient, in her phantasy, had taken the place of her mother, that is to say, she identified herself with her to such an extent that the idea of having children at the age of thirty-two had governed her unconscious life for many years. It was what psychoanalysts call one of her unconscious complexes, and the frustration of her desire became actually one of the precipitating factors of her neurosis. The fortune-teller's prophecy had evidently proved wrong, after all, but it is also true that by introducing into her " fortune " a circumstance relating to an intimate detail of her mother's life he hit upon the daughter's most ardent unconscious desire. To put it in other words, his forecast disclosed a distinct unconscious idea in the patient's mind. Freud emphasises that he could not see by what ordinary means of information the fortune-teller could have arrived at such a conclusion. On the other hand, he had no reason to doubt the *bona fides* of his patient, or to question the veracity of her account. Accordingly he had to admit that a telepathic interpretation of the case was the only one which offered a satisfactory explanation.

Freud's second observation refers again to a fortune-teller's " prophecy ". The patient, a young man, fell ill at the time of his beloved sister's marriage. In this case psychoanalysis revealed the patient's fixation on his sister. Nevertheless, he encouraged the marriage against the disapproval of their parents. It was at that time that the young man consulted a lady astrologer. The astrologer was wont to " prophesy " her client's future by means of a horoscope starting from his birth data. The young man gave her the birth data of his brother-in-law instead of his own and was told that he would die the next July or August from poisoning by crayfish or oysters.

Now, his brother-in-law did not die at the predicted time. But the fact is that he had been taken ill the previous summer, before the patient had consulted the astrologer and the cause of his illness was in actual fact poisoning from crayfish or oysters. Analysis showed that the young man had not at that time overcome his unconscious hatred of the rival who had married his sister. Hence his repressed wish that he might have died of the poisoning. In this case, too, it was quite unlikely that the astrologer could have learned by some ordinary channels of information of this insignificant detail from the life-history of the brother-in-law. Accordingly, Freud was led to assume that here, again, she had " tapped " her client's unconscious in some telepathic way.

It must be admitted that as far as proofs are concerned these observations can hardly compare with accounts of similar occurrences in the literature of psychical research. There are no confirmatory reports by two independent witnesses available, no contemporary notes taken of the incidents, etc. All we learn is based on second-hand information and largely rests on the authority of Professor Freud. However, this authority is good enough for our purpose and the flaws in the material evidence are more than made up by the deeper insight which we gain into the psychological background of the observations. Freud's analysis throws the mental attitude of the agent into sharper perspective. In the first case it is obviously his patient's preconscious wish to have children which attains telepathic activity upon the mind of another person. In the second case, it is the young man's repressed death wishes against his brother-in-law which are " sensed " by the percipient in a telepathic way. In both instances a strong emotional colouring of the ideas concerned is unmistakable. They are closely connected with the unconscious neurotic conflicts of the patients and were in fact largely responsible for their illnesses. From observations like these Freud concludes that it is emotionally emphasised complexes in their transition from the unconscious to the preconscious state which are particularly apt to assume telepathic activity. This theory is indeed in good keeping with the psychological setting in a vast number of spontaneous occurrences and has been widely quoted in the literature of psychical research.

It may, however, be argued that Freud's theory—derived as it is from neurotic patients—is valid only under abnormal conditions. Thus it may be well to put it to the test in a case of what might be called telepathy in everyday life, which occurred in my own family. It dates back to 1940 when the arrival in this country of a letter from the U.S.A. was something of a sensation, particularly when containing news from distant friends and relations. My wife had actually received such a letter from Clarence, her half-cousin, with whom she had spent a happy time in America a few years before her marriage. He, too, had married in the meantime and there was a photograph of Clarence's wife, Mathilda, attached to his letter, showing her in the company of two more ladies all unknown to my wife. She was engaged in housework and was just thinking of the photograph, while my little daughter Barbara, aged four, was absorbed in play by her side. At the very moment the child, for no apparent reason, uttered the name of *Mathilda.* I may add that this name, in its English version was quite unknown to Barbara at that time. When asked on the next day whether she remembered the name she replied : " Yes, I was having a game with mummy ".

My wife produced the following chain of associations : " No, I do not know Mathilda . . . I was wondering which one was she on the picture. I only know they had married about the same time as we did and have a child of about Barbara's age . . . and Clarence now writes that they are going to have another baby. These lucky Americans . . . they can afford such a luxury."

My wife's associations speak for themselves. They show that there was a marked emotional stress on her pre-occupation with thoughts of Mathilda. For reasons which need not be further elaborated in the present context she was identifying herself with Clarence's wife and it was obviously this attitude which provided the emotional stress which was in the last outcome responsible for the telepathic transmission of the name. Barbara's utterance was in this way a reaction comparable with what the early workers in psychical research described as a motor automatism. However this may be, the case shows that not only neurotic complexes, but emotionally emphasised ideas in any normal person may assume telepathic activity under favourable circumstances. Here, too, the method of free association may then be invoked to reveal the presence of an unconscious or pre-conscious complex as the principal conditioning factor.

Freud's theory seems to be in good keeping with the psychological background of telepathy both under normal and abnormal conditions, but the general statement that it is the repression, or emotional emphasis of a certain idea which provides the driving force of its telepathic transmission, is obviously in need of qualification. Repressed, or otherwise emotionally stressed mental processes are a regular feature of our psychic life. It is the natural background of conscious mental activity. Yet, there is nothing to indicate that unconscious mental contents invariably affect the minds of other persons in a telepathic way. Indeed, precisely the opposite is the case. Why, then, one may ask, do unconscious complexes assume telepathic activity in rare cases only, and why do they remain inactive in the overwhelming majority? And what are the psychological conditions that must be fulfilled at the receiving end of the process? What are the pre-requisities of telepathic sensitiveness on the part of the percipient? Freud's theory fails to account for this aspect of the telepathic occurrences and therefore, also, is in need of amplification.

* * *

More light upon the conditioning factors of telepathic sensitiveness is being thrown by an observation which comes from different quarters. It refers to a remarkable case of telepathic reading ability in a feeble-minded child. It was published in 1935 by Ferdinand von Neureiter, professor of forensic medicine in Riga. His book contains a detailed description of the patient from both the medical and psychological point of view and is supported by a detailed account of experiments carried out by Neureiter and his associates. The case deserves being reported here in some detail.

Professor Neureiter first learnt of Ilga K. from a letter by Dr. Kleinberger, a medical practitioner in the village of Trapene in Lithuania. " I should like to call your attention to an extremely interesting case. It is of a nine-year-old Lithuanian girl. Both her parents are alive and healthy; they are smallholders. I know the mother personally, she is a person of average intelligence, and there is no history of mental disorder or other abnormality in the family. There are two more children, an older and a younger one, both normal. The child in question was normal at birth, and seemed to develop physically in a normal manner. She was lively and sociable, but remained backward in speaking and at the age of seven or eight she had the vocabulary of a child of two. She was admitted to school at the age of eight. She managed to learn her letters but was unable to make any progress beyond that point and her teacher realised that she was suffering from a pronounced reading disability. He noticed, however, that when he was standing near the girl, reading the passage *sotto-voce*, or only in *thought* to himself, she was able to read without mistakes a context which she had never been able to read before. In fact, she could read any context required in any foreign language, although she had command of the Lithuanian language only."

Dr. Kleinberger adds that the child's number sense was equally poor, but here, too, she was able to solve the most intricate mathematical problems if the calculation was being made by the teacher mentally at the same time. Another fact reported to Dr. Kleinberger was that Ilga's mother was unable to hide anything from her child. She knew at once where the object was secreted. Dr. Kleinberger remarked that he was himself able to confirm this observation.

Professor Neureiter, after some hesitation, agreed to examine the child in collaboration with several members of the staff of the University of Riga. Part of his investigation was carried out at his residence in Riga, another part in Ilga's home, with a number of Professor Neureiter's colleagues as witnesses present. In most of the experiments Professor Neureiter himself acted as the agent. In others this part was played by Professor Brueckmann, by Dr. Kleinberger, by Ilga's little brother, aged eleven, or by her mother. As a rule, agent and percipient were placed in two separate rooms, but when they were both seated in the same room, their backs were turned to one another and they were separated by a curtain. Particular care was taken to exclude involuntary expressive movements, unconscious whispering, or other clues which might be given by the agents. A few examples may illustrate the procedure :

Professor Brueckmann writes the following calculation on a sheet of paper : $4 \cdot 4 + 5 \cdot 5 = 41$ and hands it over to Ilga's mother who is playing the part of the agent. Mrs. K. turns to Professor Neureiter, stating that she does not understand the problem. Professor Neureiter is just about to explain that the dots indicate signs of multiplication when the child, unexpectedly, utters the number 41. Obviously her mother, following Professor Neureiter's explanation, was just considering the result of the calculation sum and at that very moment the " transmission " took place.

On another occasion Neureiter's colleague, Professor Amsler, writes out a list of words and figures in an adjoining room. The list is handed to Ilga's mother who is situated behind the curtain, while Ilga, watched by the experimenters, is playing in front of the curtain. Without interrupting her game and without being asked to do so she correctly reproduces the whole list : *ger*, *til*, *tli* ; 123, 213, 312. Neureiter remarks that her voice differs on these occasions from her ordinary way of speaking. She pronounces each syllable more distinctly, in a somewhat stilted, artificial manner. In another test she produces the number 42, put down in writing by the experimenter as 12. Neureiter's reproduction of his handwriting reveals the source of this mistake. Ilga's mother mistook the 4 for a 1 which again shows that the part of the agent in this experiment was played by none but her. I may mention here that, to begin with, Ilga was only successful with her mother acting as an agent. Yet the following experiment is an instructive example of a test which met with an initial failure but was followed by a success. Neureiter reports : " I take the place of the agent and try to transmit to the child the figures 9 and 2 ; then a sentence printed in a Lithuanian primer : *Mate Gaja uz leti*. I concentrate hard upon my task, stressing every syllable in thought . . . yet in spite of all my effort the percipient remains silent. I am just on the point to close the book and to break off the experiment with some disappointment when my eye is caught by the word *Brute* (bride) in the context of a Lithuanian poem, the first words of which I was trying in vain to transmit. And at that very moment the child, situated in the adjoining room, produced the word. This was apparently the best way to promote the telepathic transmission, although—or rather because—I refrained from intentional sending." And he adds by way of a footnote : " When I noticed the word *Brute* I wondered why it was used in a modern Lithuanian first spelling book. It was a foreign word, derived from the German *Braut* and obsolete at that. There was, instead, the genuine Lithuanian word *Ligava* available which would have better suited its purpose. These were the thoughts that were passing through my mind while I did not in any case think of my original aim."

Another type of experiment followed the pattern of the popular parlour room game of looking for a hidden object. Dr. Kleinberger hid his watch under one of the cushions on a couch while Ilga was staying in the adjoining room. On entering she exclaims at once : " The watch is under the cushions ". On this occasion it took her some time to find it and she had to turn up every cushion in order to produce the watch.

However, her most spectacular performance was at what we described as telepathic reading. The tests confirm that she was able to reproduce fluently any passage read by her mother, whether it was written in Lithuanian, in German, in English, French or even Latin. When she was reading in a foreign language she made the mistakes which were in keeping with her mother's level of education. She read numbers in a French context in the Lithuanian language, mispronounced French words or technical terms in the same way, etc. On several occasions she was equally successful with other persons playing the part of the agent.

The medical examination of the child revealed no abnormalities. Her photograph shows a somewhat dull looking girl with a broad skull and coarse features. No stigmata seem to be present. Neureiter reports that she took an intelligent interest in her surroundings, showed marked dexterity at manual tasks, played with toys, was able to run errands and to obey orders. He had her intelligence tested by an educational psychologist. She performed poorly on both the Binet-Simon and the Buehler-Hetzer scale, reaching the mental age of a child of approximately four years and an I.Q. of forty-two. However, her most pronounced disability was at reading in the "ordinary way". She was able to recognise a few isolated letters only and failed to read even the simplest words. By contrast, she could write fairly well, copied handwriting and print correctly, but was again unable to read her own handwriting. The specimen reproduced in Neureiter's book shows mistakes of so-called agraphic character, coupled with a tendency to reverse letters.

The combination of Ilga's reading disability with the ability to write is of special interest in the present connection. It suggests the presence in her case of what neurologists describe as congenital word-blindness or alexia. Little is known regarding the causation of this defect but it is generally assumed that it is due to a specific disorder on the plane of the highest visual functions, due perhaps to impairment of the cerebral cortex in the left angular region. Patients suffering from this disability are not blind ; they can see well ; they can distinguish the shapes of objects ; they can appreciate pictures ; but written words convey no meaning to them : they are word-blind.

Ilga's striking telepathic reading ability gains added significance in the light of these findings. She is unable to read, but has developed what appears as an unusual telepathic sensitiveness to words read by other persons. There is an unmistakable correspondence between these two things. Her specific defect and her specific ability dovetail with one another and the latter might well be described as the result of a tendency to make up for her original shortcoming, that is to say, as a tendency to compensate for a functional inferiority in a way well known to biologists and psychologists in both the organic and psychological sphere.

An observation of my own in the field proper of neurology may illustrate the point. In 1929 I described a case of an elderly patient who developed the clinical picture of so-called pure word-blindness on the basis of cerebral sclerosis. His symptoms showed far-reaching similarity with Ilga's congenital defect. But in his case there was a peculiar fluctuation of symptoms which attracted our interest. On certain days he was able to recognise at least a few short syllables ; on other days his alexia was complete and he was unable to decipher even a few isolated letters.

It is needless to say that this patient failed to display any unusual tendency to compensation such as was observed in Ilga K., but he showed another peculiarity. Though utterly unable to read in the usual way on his bad days, he was able to recognise isolated letters and syllables written on his skin.

Conversely, any temporary improvement of his visual reading ability, observed on his good days, was coupled with an impairment or even loss of ability to read by the skin. In other words : the temporary improvement of his tactile or kinaesthetic function seemed to take place at the expense of his residual visual functions and, *vice versa*, the deterioration of his residual reading ability seemed to result in an increased acuity of his tactile and kinaesthetic perceptions.

This type of compensation is in fact a familiar feature of the physiology of the senses. Remarkable examples of hyperaesthesia of hearing or of touch have repeatedly been described in blind persons. It is proverbial in bats. We may also recall that one of the early theories of telepathy actually sought to explain, or to explain away, telepathy by reference to an unusual degree of sensory hyperaesthesia. The same idea is reflected in the various legends of blind seers or prophets from ancient times. It will be noted, however, that in the familiar instances of sensory hyperfunction the assumed compensation tendency is confined to the ordinary sensory level only, and there is nothing to indicate that telepathy or clairvoyance is more frequent in blind or otherwise incapacitated persons than in ordinary people. In any case, attempts to make the institutions for the blind or for the deaf a happy hunting ground for psychical research have so far proved a failure.

Ilga's case is in this way unique of its kind. She is neither blind nor does she possess any extraordinary degree of sensory hyperaesthesia. Accordingly, any theory seeking to explain her unusual ability by reference to a compensation tendency of the familiar kind must admit that this tendency works in a rather unorthodox way. There is only one point in which Neureiter's observation seems to conform with laws familiar in the field of biology and psychology in general : this is the peculiar correspondence between Ilga's specific defect or minus-function on the one hand and her specific ability or hyperfunction on the other. It is this peculiar correspondence that gives a clue to at least a tentative hypothesis of the conditioning factors which may be operative on the part of a telepathic percipient. It suggests that telepathic sensitiveness may be due to compensation for some kind of deficiency on the higher cognitive levels, and that in certain cases the specific nature of this sensitiveness may be conditioned by the specific nature of the existing defect.

Here again, as in the case of Freud's hypothesis regarding the psychology of the agent, a number of objections can be raised. It may be argued that Ilga's case is too rare to permit any valid generalisations ; that she is a mental defective, suffering from a specific disability, whereas telepathy has been observed in otherwise perfectly sane and well-balanced individuals. Before we can enter into a discussion of these objections it will be as well to consider a few more cases from which additional light may be thrown on the problem of telepathic sensitiveness.

Professor William Brown, in his article on *Psychology and Psychical Research*, briefly describes an observation of this kind. One of his patients awakening from hypnosis, reported to him that while he was lying on the couch " the vivid picture of a page of a scientific journal appeared to him with two columns in form of a letter signed at the bottom ". On reflection, Dr. Brown realised that while the patient was in the hypnotic state his own eye had been caught by one of the letters printed in a copy of *Nature* that lay in front of him. There was no " normal " means by which the patient could have caught a glance of the page in question. Dr. Brown handed the copy of *Nature* to him. The patient looked through it and, to quote Professor Brown's own words, found " the identical letter ".

A great number of similar observations of telepathy in the hypnotic state, some of them equally well authenticated as Professor Brown's case, have been described in the literature. Their relevance to our problem is obvious. It is common ground that the hypnotic state implies an impairment of the higher strata of consciousness, in conjunction with mental dissociation. We have to assume that such telepathic sensitiveness as can be observed in this condition is due to the operation of a similar compensation tendency as is involved in the case of an impairment of certain cognitive functions on the organic level. On the other hand, the emergence of unusual hyperfunctions involving memory or other special abilities is a well-known feature of the hypnotic state. I need only mention the striking examples of unconscious time-appreciation, of creative activities, etc., in hypnotised persons.

If this be true, Dr. Brown's observation essentially follows the pattern of our previous case, although with certain points of difference. First, the minus-function (that is, the impairment of consciousness), was transient in his patient. It will be noted, however, that so was his telepathic sensitiveness. Secondly, the impairment of his consciousness was all-round or global, as compared with the more circumscribed nature of the disability in Ilga's case. Accordingly, his telepathic sensitiveness was not confined to a single function, but covered a somewhat broader field. We shall see on a later page that, *mutatis mutandis*, the same considerations apply to telepathic occurrences in dreams and in the mediumistic trance. But here, again, it will be as well to cast a glance at cases of less spectacular type, such as occur under conditions of everyday life, and to examine how far they can be explained in the light of our theory.

The following observation is one of the few instances in which I myself was playing the part of a telepathic percipient, whilst my daughter, aged eight, at that time, played the part of the agent. She was looking at the illustration to a story in the *Sunday Express* which had " nothing to do with the war ". It was the picture of the horse, Peter, that attracted her attention. It was a dull Sunday morning, about 11 o'clock, when she suddenly turned to me : " What do you think, daddy, how old is this horse ? " I was little interested in Peter, the horse, and threw only a very perfunctory look at the picture, but without a moment's hesitation I remarked in a jocular way : " It is 17 ". The fact is that in the caption the horse's age was given as 17. The probability of my having guessed his correct age by mere chance is obviously very slight ; on the other hand, I had not even seen the paper on that day, so that sensory leakage can safely be ruled out of the question. The only reasonable explanation is telepathy from Barbara to myeslf.

In this case a variety of factors can be invoked to account for my reaction. The night before, I had taken part in a banquet at L. and had consumed a quantity of drinks far in excess of my moderate capacity, and I had awakened with a slight headache. This alone might well account for something like a minus-function on my part. But there is another side to my experiences on the previous night. It was a convivial bachelors' party with easy-going gaiety culminating in community singing in which I joined, much against my habit. I cannot, for obvious reasons, discuss here the bearing of this experience upon my attitude towards the group, towards various aspects of social life, etc. The problem will be dealt with from a more general point of view in a later chapter. But however this may be, it can well be assumed that the episode described entailed something like a temporarily loosened self-control on my part and that this had furnished an additional contributing factor towards my unusual role as a telepathic percipient.

Summing up, the necessary conditioning factors of telepathy in a concrete case can be described as follows. They are constituted of two complementary sets of conditions, one concerning the attitude of the agent, the other the attitude of the percipient. On the part of the agent we pointed to the presence of repression, total or partial, or to a pronounced emotional stress of certain thoughts, ideas or complexes. On the part of the percipient we found what we described as a minus-function in the physiological or psychological sphere, lasting or transient, global or circumscribed, as the common denominator of the cases reviewed. To this we must add as a third factor the tendency to compensate for the existing minus-function or defect, whether this tendency be the outcome of slackened control, of released activity of lower mental strata, or of the otherwise unimpaired general vitality of the person concerned.

It is clear that a constellation governed by such a multiplicity of factors is unlikely to occur on more than a few extraordinary occasions. Ilga K.'s striking telepathic reading ability is one of the rare examples of this kind. Not only did her clinical picture present the requisite blend of conditioning factors, but it was persistent enough to permit their closer investigation. In the rest of the examples discussed here, the general setting is less favourable for such an examination, but in rough outline it is likewise suggestive of the presence of identical psychological and physiological conditions. It is readily understood that there may exist all conceivable shades of transition from the ideal set of conditioning factors to equivocal or utterly negative ones. There may be cases in which the whole situation would favour telepathy on the part of a would-be percipient, but in which, in the absence of a suitable agent, telepathy would fail to materialise. This, for instance, was the case in some of the unsuccessful experiments with Ilga K. Again, there may be a would-be agent who fails to meet, half-way as it were, a suitable percipient. For instance, we may visualise a psychological constellation in which Barbara's mother would be pondering about Mathilda's photograph, with Mrs. Smith or Mrs. Jones by her side, instead of Barbara. Or else, we may contemplate Barbara, thrilled with the picture of the veteran horse, whilst her father is restored to his normal self after the experience of the previous night : in both instances it is unlikely that telepathy would have taken place.

But we have reason to focus our interest on as foolproof and unequivocal cases as we can possibly find, however rare they may be. An eclipse of the sun may be an event just as rare as a case of congenital word-blindness, coupled with an unusual tendency to its compensation. Yet there can be little doubt that it has been the study of such unusual occurrences as a solar eclipse which astronomy owed much of its advance at the beginning of its career. It may well be that the few firmly established cases of spontaneous telepathy which can be subjected to closer scrutiny are going to play a similar part in the history of psychical research.

It can rightly be asked, however, whether the principles derived from sporadic observations like these can be applied to the vast group of laboratory experiments with telepathy. Under laboratory conditions the whole mental setting is evidently entirely different. It lacks the spontaneity of real life. Things are expected to happen according to plan and they are actually made to happen to a pre-arranged schedule. Accordingly they can hardly possess the same emotional relevance to the minds of the agent or the percipient as real happenings. And what actually are the things that are made to happen under laboratory condition ? The agent looks at the card symbol, puts the card down, records its name, casts a short glance at the next one, puts down its name in writing, etc. Again, the percipient, on receiving a signal from the experimenter, registers his guess, waits for the next signal, again registers his guess, waits for the next signal, and so on and so forth. Many subjects have complained of the monotonous nature of this procedure, especially if it stretches over a period of days, weeks, or even months.

However, on reading Dr. Rhine's description of his earlier tests the picture is different. He stresses the importance of the right atmosphere, of a free, cordial relationship between the experimenter and his subject, between agent and percipient. Observers who had the opportunity of witnessing his experiments were greatly impressed with Rhine's personality with " his striking combination of humane sympathy with a most single minded devotion to truth ". This spirit, says Professor McDougall in his Foreword to Dr. Rhine's book on E.S.P., he succeeded in conferring on his collaborators, creating " an important, perhaps indispensable, condition of the striking successes reported ".

There can be no doubt that the personality of the experimenter as the leader of the group may profoundly affect the outcome of the tests. In the previous chapter I pointed to the significance of what I called telepathic leakage or para-experimental telepathy in experiments of this class. It is clear that, if the subject is suitable for E.S.P. at all, the experimenter's unconscious wishes and expectations may well be able to influence results, to promote an attitude favouring success or conducive to failure. This, for instance, is illustrated by S. G. Soal's failure to duplicate Rhine's successful experiments with Mrs. Eileen Garrett, the English medium. On the other hand, it will be recalled that Soal himself was highly successful in a series of experiments suggesting a new aspect of extra-sensory perception, i.e. precognitive telepathy.

Mr. G. N. M. Tyrrell throws another interesting sidelight upon the psychological conditions obtaining in experiments of the Duke type. I mentioned his mechanical apparatus for testing E.S.P. faculty. It consisted originally of five upholstered black boxes placed behind a screen. The agent, unobserved by the percipient, puts a pointer into one of the boxes and the percipient registers his guess over a series of many hundreds of trials. Tyrrell, describing this procedure, remarks that even with his most successful subject, Miss G. I., high extra-chance results were confined to short runs or *bursts* only, alternating with phases in which her scores were of chance nature only. In Miss G. I.'s words, these lucky spells were accompanied by a " peculiar and rather exalted feeling in which she felt that it was almost impossible to fail ". Her attitude during these periods reminded Mr. Tyrrell of a trance-like state with mental dissociation. But he suggests at the same time that they were invariably associated with conditions of physical and mental well-being and were broken by any sign of indisposition. Otherwise the psychological side of the picture is obscure. Psychoanalysts may be inclined to comment on the possible unconscious significance to agent or percipient of the black boxes or of the ominous pointer device. But it is clear that in so doing they would venture on the treacherous ground of unwarranted speculation.

However this may be, it is obvious that no hypothesis framed in such general terms as have been formulated so far can do justice to the peculiar erratic distribution pattern of failure and success in mass experiments. Moreover, it can be argued that most of the materials used are even less likely to possess any emotional appeal to the experimenter or his subjects than Mr. Tyrrell's pointer device or upholstered black boxes. We have only to recall the geometrical symbols printed on the Zener cards used in hundreds of thousands of card-calling tests. On the other hand, the possibility that such arid symbols may nevertheless happen to be registered by the percipient in a moment of absent-mindedness or mental dissociation, favouring telepathic sensitiveness to precisely the item in question, cannot be ruled out. Further, there may be short periods when a particular symbol may become charged with some evanescent feeling tone conditioned by a passing mood of the agent. Such moods may pass unnoticed by all those participating in the experiments, but their cumulative effect may suffice to tip the balance in favour of highly significant extra-chance scores in a given series of tests.

Indirect clues pointing in this direction are furnished by the following experiments. I asked a number of subjects to glance at one of the Zener cards and to tell me their impressions. A former patient of mine, a lady of forty-six, was shown the " five squares ". She exclaimed : " Oh, they are like a repulsive face staring at me ! " In a similar vein, the " wavy lines " reminded her of " disgusting little worms ". A child of seven associated the " five crosses " with kisses in a letter, whilst her mother found they reminded her of the melancholy array of soldier's graves. There were other subjects whose associations were less imaginative and colourful. But the few reactions of the imaginative type are sufficient to show that even such trivial items as geometrical figures, wavy lines or plus signs, may call forth a wealth of emotionally coloured imagery in suitable subjects. The vast body of experience derived from the Rorschach test go far to confirm this proposition.

But if this is true it is fair to assume that the identical imagery may be looming at the back of their minds when the same subjects take part in E.S.P. tests with the same materials. It may then provide the hidden source of at least part of the emotional charge which, we said, may be responsible for extra-chance scoring even under the most uninspiring laboratory conditions.

It may be argued at this point that the more imaginative subjects in my association-tests were nothing but willing tools in my hands, obliging me, as they did, with producing precisely the associations which I wanted them to produce. This may indeed have been the case. But, if so, it only confirms our thesis of the importance of unconscious suggestions—telepathic or otherwise—acting from the experimenter upon his subject and influencing his reactions. We only have to replace one experimental situation with the other in order to realise that similar imponderable factors may account for either failure or success in an experiment deliberately designed as telepathic.

It would be idle to pursue this chain of reasoning any further. It is only apt to lead us too far afield in the sphere of speculation, unwarranted by factual observations. We must reconcile ourselves to the fact that the method of mass experiments is incapable of yielding deeper insight into the minds of the agent and the percipient and that what information we can extract regarding the psychological background of these experiments is essentially derived from the few well-established spontaneous cases which we have discussed so far.

Chapter IV

COMPARATIVE ANALYSIS AND THE SCATTER THEORY

Our vindication of the study of spontaneous occurrences, as opposed to experiments in psychical research may seem to entail a contradiction to the prevailing trend of the new science. Contemporary psychical research justly prides itself with having outgrown the stage when it relied chiefly on anecdotal accounts of a few spectacular occurrences by untrained observers and compiled by a group of amateur investigators. We have seen that it has gone far towards establishing beyond any doubt the existence of psi-phenomena and towards raising their investigation to the standard of repeatable and mathematically assessable laboratory experiments.

This should not, however, obscure the limitations of an exclusively quantitative approach. The compilation of data, no matter how solid and unassailable, does not by itself constitute a science, and it may well be questioned whether they can claim to be the " stubborn and irreducible facts " which, in the words of William James, are the first prerequisites of the scientific method. Clearly, psychical research by confining its attention to phenomena which pass through the sieve of the statistician and by discarding the remainder as irrelevant, would arrive at a one-sided—if not distorted—picture of the available evidence which may bar the way for any further progress for years to come.

We described how Rhine and his followers started from the notion of a possible transmission in some extra-sensory way of well-defined perceptual images or sensory impressions. It is fair to say that Rhine himself has never professed to accept this hypothesis without qualification. But it is still tacitly implied in the attitude of many workers in psychical research. However, in adopting such a working hypothesis, the experimenter is easily led to the totally unwarranted view that paranormal cognition is really concerned with a quasi-sensory perception of distinct sense-data or their psychological representations. Such a conception is certainly not borne out by the facts. It is partly due to the difficulty of describing the phenomena in an unbiased manner, partly to our habit of conceiving of mental processes in terms of an obsolete atomistic theory, and lastly to the experimenter's deliberate choice in confining his inquiry to artificially simplified and mathematically treatable material. It will be recalled that the materials used, and the reactions recorded, in the experimental situation are strictly selective. The subject must comply with the conditions chosen and with the rules prescribed. If pure telepathy is being investigated the percipient has the choice among the mental pictures of five geometrical symbols previously agreed upon by the participants. He has to concentrate on these symbols to the exclusion of any other idea that may pass through his mind. A fairly large proportion of subjects has indeed scored striking results under such conditions. That is to say, they were able to score hits at the mental pictures selected by the agent in a significant number of trials and thus to satisfy the experimenter that telepathy had taken place. The same is true for experiments of the pre-cognitive, clairvoyant, or mixed clairvoyant and telepathic type, and to a lesser degree even for Whately Carington's experiments with telepathic drawings. But it is clear that such a procedure can hardly yield results other than were already anticipated by the experimenter. In the extreme case his attitude towards his subjects would bear a considerable resemblance to the way in which a vindictive police constable extracts information from a culprit, leaving him no alternative between the answers " Yes " or " No " and little chance to tell the rest of his story which might elucidate the real state of affairs.

It is true to say that such an insistence on two, and only two, alternative reactions is one of the prerequisites of the statistical method. Whenever the experimenter makes allowance for the possibility of other interpretations he is up against the difficulty of assessing the correctness, or otherwise, of an infinite variety of possible answers, none of which may be totally wrong or totally right in a strictly scientific sense. But the fact is, that the infinite variety of thought and emotion, of meaning and purpose that constitute mental life is fundamentally inaccessible to quantitative treatment. It cannot be summed up in terms of cut and dried "elements" in the minds of an agent and a percipient whose congruity or incongruity can either be asserted or denied with the exactitude of an unequivocal mathematical statement. Moreover, it is clear that outside the prearranged experimental situation the very statement of their congruity or correspondence is itself in need of definition.

It will be recalled that in most spontaneous occurrences which we described on earlier pages the claimed correspondence between an idea in the mind of an agent and a percipient was of a peculiar, indirect, symbolic or metaphorical nature. In many instances the correspondence is suggested by the correlations which exist between the whole and the part, between the essential and the accidental, between a distinct idea and a far-fetched association which is connected with it, between the real thing and its symbolic representation. This is well illustrated by some of Warcollier's observations which we have quoted. We mentioned the experiment in which he tried telepathically to convey the picture of an airship moored in an aerodrome, and in which his percipient drew a number of ladders leaning against a wall. On analysis he found that the telepathic copy was a reproduction of the lateral supports of the aerodrome and left out the more essential parts of the original. Or we may recall the experiment of Professor Gilbert Murray in which the agent thought of a passage from a novel by Dostojevsky and in which the percipient received the impression of the "Russian atmosphere", but failed to reproduce the item in question. Innumerable examples of the same kind could be quoted from the literature. More recently Dr. R. H. Thouless emphasised that symbolic representation as opposed to photographic likeness of reproduction is a fundamental feature of telepathy, and described a series of experiments illustrating this point.

However, it is clear that the appreciation of correlations of this type cannot be achieved along strictly mathematical lines; it is a matter of subjective interpretation. This precisely is one of the main reasons why Rhine and his school rejected altogether the evidence of spontaneous phenomena and resorted to the method of mass experiments. However, we emphasised that a one-sided approach to measurable and calculable data is apt to disregard an important part of reality ; the one which refuses to submit to such a method. It eliminates many of the vagaries and imponderables of psychological processes, but in so doing it empties out the baby with the bath, as it were, and defeats its own purpose. On the other hand, it cannot be denied that unless we define the principles of a non-mathematical approach to our problem there will remain a strong case in favour of the method developed by Rhine and his followers, whatever its limitations.

It is a remarkable fact that the early workers largely failed to pay due attention to the problem of method. They were chiefly concerned with the accumulation of facts. They laid down certain rules which had to be observed, certain conditions to which an incident described had to conform before its authenticity was taken for granted. For instance, it was emphasised that the observation concerned should be recorded in writing, or communicated to some other person as soon as practicable, and in any case before the percipient could gain knowledge by normal means of the event to which his experience corresponded. Special emphasis was laid on written statements signed and countersigned by two independent witnesses, or on other contemporaneous documentary evidence. These safeguards were certainly indispensable for the establishment of the factual evidence of the case and to satisfy the sceptical general public. But it will be noted that they give no lead regarding the psychological assessment of the material, no standard by which to gauge the telepathic or non-telepathic nature of the occurrence.

Many recorded observations both by students of psychical research and medical psychologists up to our days show the difficulties which arise from such a state of affairs. The following example quoted from a recent article on *Telepathy in Dreams* by N. Fodor illustrates the point : One night the author dreamt that he was president of the world. The same night his wife had a dream that she was Queen Alexandra of England. Fodor suggests that there is a telepathic correspondence between these two dreams. But he extended his inquiry to a dream by his daughter on the same night. This dream need not be reproduced here in detail. The point is that in Fodor's view the psychoanalytic interpretation of the latter also bore striking resemblance to his own and his wife's dreams and contained a reference to the idea of a God-like father, the ruler of the world.

Now, the suggested Freudian reading of these dreams may be fully justified and a close resemblance of their latent meanings undeniable. But does this resemblance (or even identity) of meaning warrant their telepathic interpretation? Paul Schilder, on reviewing similar observations published in the psychoanalytical literature, has criticised the attitude of the authors towards this crucial problem and warned them against being misled by the equivocal language of the unconscious. The deeper we descend in the symbolic sphere, he contends, the greater is the similarity between the thoughts of various persons, although it would be rash to ascribe this similarity to telepathy. Evidently, this objection is only too true with regard to Fodor's examples.

The same argument applies to some of the instances which are described in Dr. L. Bendit's book on *Paranormal Cognition*. In Case 1 he describes how during a session of psychotherapy with one of his patients he himself was seized by a sudden wave of unmotivated anxiety. The patient had just been speaking about her own neurotic fears of Hell fire without, however, showing any evidence of emotion. When questioned, she confessed that she had on her part been "panicking" during their conversation. Bendit assumes that in this case he had been "invaded" by his patient's neurotic fear in some telepathic way.

In this instance, too, a telepathic interpretation is undoubtedly suggestive. But here, again, the author would hardly be able to convince a sceptic. How can he prove that his fear did not spring from the same unconscious source as the fear of his patient? And, even if we dismiss this surmise, how can he prove that their common experiences were really identical, and due to telepathic correspondence? Rhine has pointed out that the student of psychical research dealing with spontaneous phenomena has nothing but his common-sense judgment to rely on and that this in turn is apt to vary with "the common sense (or bias) of the person making the judgment".

What method, other than the quantitative experiment and

its statistical evaluation, is then at our disposal? Clearly, it must be a method which is congenial to the phenomena and which at the same time complies with the requirements of a rational scientific approach. It must be based on a clear notion: (1) of what we mean by telepathic correspondence, (2) of what we mean by thoughts, ideas or other mental elements whose telepathic correspondence we assert, and (3) on an understanding regarding the criteria on which the statement that their apparent similarity is not due to chance alone is based.

From such spontaneous occurrences as were reviewed on previous pages a few principles emerge which can serve as a basis for further discussion. First, we pointed out that the claimed correspondence must refer to things on the purely mental plane, that is to say, to thoughts, ideas or other elements or motifs in the minds of two persons. Failing this, the experience concerned cannot legitimately be described as a case of pure telepathy. This is, however, a largely academic qualification and it will be remembered that it was introduced chiefly in view of the primarily psychological orientation of our inquiry.

Secondly, the thought, or idea, which is claimed to be reproduced in a telepathic way must be identifiable as a distinct mental element: this is certainly a matter of subjective interpretation, viz. of an essentially psychological approach, and may therefore appear somewhat arbitrary to a zealous advocate of the quantitative method. But it will be noted that precisely the same problem arises when the scientist refers to an isolated "system", as distinct from the "remainder of things in the Universe" (Whitehead), or to "observables" (L. Bragg), which are the ultimate facts upon which his argument is based. The fact is that the isolation of systems or observables in the physical world is a procedure by no means less arbitrary than the isolation of elements or motifs in the psychological field. However, both are indispensable prerequisites of our orientation in the world, failing which no further argument and no science, physical or psychological, is conceivable.

Thirdly, the element or motif thus isolated from the rest of the mental content, must contain a sufficient number of distinctive features. Failing this the objection of chance coincidence could hardly be dismissed even though the item in question may be reproduced in great detail. It is true that the telepathic reproduction of a multiplicity of features is a rare event and cannot be expected as a general rule. But it goes without saying that it is precisely this criterion which may decide the merits of a concrete case.

A last feature that needs careful consideration is the assumed temporal coincidence of the two mental events under review. Temporal coincidence is tacitly implied in every case of alleged telepathy. But here, too, little attention has been paid to the necessity of clarifying its meaning. We will return to this question on a later page. Here it will be sufficient to note that temporal coincidence or simultaneousness is an elastic notion in the psychological sphere. It cannot be defined by reference to the positions of the hands of two clocks. It can only be expressed by referring to things on the purely mental plane, i.e. to two co-existing series of psychological processes in the minds of two separate persons. But what is the criterion of their "co-existence"? Clearly, co-existence of the two series can reasonably be assumed whenever they are of topical interest, conscious or unconscious, to those concerned; it is a function of their vital significance at a given moment to the persons experiencing them. But it is readily understood that this question can only be decided on the ground of a careful psychological analysis which is not confined to superficial strata but which probes deep into the hidden psychological implications of the item in question. In short, in order to arrive at the notion of temporal coincidence in the psychological sphere we have to extend our inquiry to the remotest folds of the personality, covering the whole field of the experiences of both agent and percipient. This procedure may be called a method of comparative analysis of the total psychological situation in which we presume that telepathy is taking place.

This brings us to a crucial point of our inquiry. It shows that for a variety of reasons the approach most appropriate to our issue is of an essentially psychological nature; it is, in effect, nothing else than a modified method of psychoanalysis, applied to two or more persons instead of to one, and with its compass extended so as to comprise a new factor, the telepathic, entering the picture.

It may be objected at this juncture that the extension of our frame of reference to such a highly complex psychological situation may still more increase the risks attending the orthodox analytical method. These risks have already been anticipated by Schilder's critical remarks and were exemplified by Fodor's analysis of alleged telepathic dreams. However, this does not by itself detract from the potential value of the method. It only underlines the dangers of probing too far into the ambiguous depths of the unconscious, of psychoanalytical over-interpretation whose results may be falsified by the very sensitiveness of the method. Otherwise, the method of comparative analysis, if only applied with the necessary discretion, has both the same merit and shortcomings as any other method which is being used by contemporary psychology. No method is able to dispense altogether with the factor of subjective interpretation, whether it be concerned with the mind of an anxiety neurotic, with the intelligence quotient of a mentally defective or with a person's dark adaptation curve measured by optical instruments.

Summing up, the psychological approach to the problem of telepathy can rightly claim a status equal to that of the quantitative statistical method. The method of mass experiments and their mathematical evaluation furnishes the bare facts. It presents measurable and calculable data. It makes the existence of paranormal cognition an indisputable bedrock truth. But it is also true to say that it gives little insight into the nature of the phenomena and into the mental setting of an individual case. It is at this point that the investigation of sporadic occurrences by what we described as the method of comparative analysis has to step in. The significance of this class of occurrences does not lie in their limited evidential value. They permit us to focus our attention on a more detailed picture of a concrete case, they throw it into sharper perspective; they fill the gaps left between the facts established by the laboratory methods and link them up with the main body of our established psychological experience. The quantitative and the qualitative methods are in this way complementary, not mutually exclusive. They are called upon, each in turn, to make their specific contribution to the new science, and it is clear that only by the joint consideration of their findings can we arrive at a balanced picture of " all the facts " as an indispensable prerequisite of valid scientific generalisations.

It would be premature to put forward any further claims regarding the efficiency of the analytical method at this point of our argument. The proof of the pudding lies in the eating, and it will be in the subsequent parts of this book that the comparative approach as outlined here will be put to the test. But on looking back on the field covered so far, we can see that our approach has already gone far towards bridging the gulf which exists between spontaneous and experimental telepathy. In particular, we may recall two points which we made in the previous chapters. First, we showed that at bottom the same emotional factors and minus-states—organic or functional—as are involved in a sporadic case can be revealed in otherwise trifling experimental occurrences. Secondly, we emphasised that, especially in the most successful series of mass experiments it may be the experimenter's emotionally coloured attitude towards his tests, his unconscious wishes and expectations, which provide, unawares, the hidden emotional forces which account for extra chance scoring by his subjects. They may in fact, largely determine the quality of the results obtained. We shall have to revert to the role of so-called para-experimental telepathy in the further course of our argument.

There is also a third aspect of telepathy upon which our approach may throw fresh light : the problem of pre-cognitive telepathy. This is, perhaps, one of the most intriguing aspects of paranormal cognition and certainly too involved a matter to be tackled by way of an appendix to a short chapter primarily concerned with questions of method. Indeed, the problem of pre-cognitive telepathy is so intimately connected with a variety of highly technical, philosophical and metaphysical questions that I fully share the fear of " rushing in where angels fear to tread " which Whately Carington expressed in one of his recent papers dealing with this problem. But on the other hand, we shall presently see that the relevance of our findings upon this issue is so obvious that it cannot be by-passed at the present juncture. We pointed out that the very essence of the comparative analytical approach lies in its appreciation of the indirect, metaphorical nature of telepathic correspondence. We said that the percipient in spontaneous cases rarely reproduces the whole of the agent's mental content. More often than not, he seems to slip from the central idea on to its fringe, from the essential to the accidental, from the real thing to its symbolic representation. His response is not a photographic replica but rather a coded cipher representing the original. In many cases it has first to be de-coded through deep-psychological analysis before its true meaning can be understood. To put it in other words: measured by the standards of successful experiments in paranormal cognition the percipient seldom hits a bull's eye in conditions of ordinary life. He scores " near misses " scattered around the target idea of the agent. Figuratively speaking, this reaction can well be described as a deviation in the dimension of space, as it were, or as a tendency to spatial scatter.

It will, however, be as well to realise that this tendency to spatial scatter is only a very crude description of what is actually taking place. The percipient's score does not in reality deviate in what can appropriately be expressed in terms of a three-dimensional space. His hits or misses refer to things on the purely mental plane, they are not concerned with pointer-readings of the physicists, but with fleeting associations passing through his and the percipient's mind respectively which emerge from the pre-conscious or unconscious sphere for a short while before they slip back into the unknown from whence they came. Henri Bergson has rightly pointed out that to describe these psychological processes in spatialised terms is little more than a figure of speech, largely determined by the current spatialised concepts of the working of our mind.

The fact is, that whenever we pay due attention to the unconscious background of our mental life we soon come to realise that the temporal factor cannot possibly be disregarded even in the crudest diagrammatic conception of mental processes. The question of *when* is certainly of greater significance than the question of *where*.

This point may be illustrated by what elsewhere I described as an instance of *Telepathy in Macbeth*.

All hail Macbeth ! hail to thee, Thane of Glamis !
All hail Macbeth ! hail to thee, Thane of Cawdor !
All hail Macbeth, that shalt be king hereafter . . .

thus greet the Weird Sisters Macbeth on the Blasted Heath. On the ground of the telepathy hypothesis it can well be argued that the Weird Sisters, in foretelling Macbeth's rise to power, were in actual fact sensitive to his own unconscious wishes : to his desire to become Thane of Glamis, Thane of Cawdor and " king hereafter ". He first rejects this idea but soon yields to the suggestion

Whose horrid image doth unfix my hair
And make my seated heart knock at my ribs.

If this be true, the witches' forecast reflects his own sinister thoughts which were at that time looming at the back of his mind. It would be at bottom a telepathic reaction. But even if we accept the telepathic interpretation of their prophecy, it would be difficult to prove that the latter and Macbeth's unconscious desires were strictly " simultaneous " in the chronological sense. In fact we pointed out that as a general rule such an assertion can hardly be made in the psychological sphere. In any case, the witches' utterance can be interpreted in two alternative ways. It can be taken as a telepathic response to an unformulated idea, to a germ of purpose, which lay dormant in Macbeth's unconscious at that time, or else as a real anticipation of his future plans—provided that we are prepared at all to allow for such a possibility. But one thing is clear in either case : their utterance, striking though it may be, implies a deviation in time rather than in space, and can more legitimately be described in terms of a temporal, than of a spatial, scatter even though it lies in the nature of our case that it is impossible to decide whether it is then to be taken as an instance of post-cognitive or pre-cognitive telepathy in the sense of modern psychical research. On a later page we will quote an example of telepathy in a patient suffering from a schizophrenic psychosis which confronts us with precisely the same problem and it is readily understood that many cases of alleged veridical dreams may be amenable to similar alternative interpretations.

However this may be, what might be described as a tendency to spatio-temporal scatter is obviously a fundamental feature of telepathic phenomena in general. But if this is true, the striking observations of post-cognitive and pre-cognitive telepathy suggested by the Whately Carington and Soal-Goldney experiments have at least one characteristic in common with familiar occurrences of telepathy in ordinary life, and fall into an intelligible pattern. Considering the intrinsic scatter-tendency of telepathic guesses, the incidence of pre-cognitive or post-cognitive reactions is precisely what might be expected as an alternative to a bull's eye under conditions of the usual card-calling tests. On the face of it, it may even be claimed that there is no fundamental difference between "ordinary" and pre-cognitive telepathy and that what difference there may appear to exist is largely due to differences in the experimental situation, of the materials used, and of the methods of interpretation and assessment applied. It may be argued that unless the percipient in card-calling tests scores a bull's eye he cannot help slipping on to one of the cards either preceding or following the target card. Similarly, it may be pointed out, that on the ground of the scatter theory it is only to be expected that a participant in Whately Carington's drawing tests may occasionally score on either the previous or the following days' original, instead of reproducing the drawing prepared on the same day.

However, there is an important feature in which the observations of pre-cognitive telepathy seem to be in flagrant contradiction to our original assumption and to the current scientific world picture in general. So far, our argument has been based on the conception of a scatter, spatial or temporal, of the percipient's guesses, clustered around the central idea of the agent. That is to say, we made provisions for a displacement of scores from the conscious into the pre-conscious or unconscious sphere. We allowed for associations being side-tracked to forgotten items in the agent's memory, or on to unformulated thoughts which cast their shadows in the percipient's mind *ahead* of time. But in any case we only provided for telepathic sensitiveness to such items as are at the present moment, or as have been for some time past, in existence in the mind of some person, and we made no provision for the possibility that the range of telepathic sensitiveness might extend to such mental processes as have not at the time of the percipient registering his impression taken place in the agent's mind—or anywhere else. But this extension to future events actually took place in the Whately Carington and Soal-Goldney experiments or, if the evidence of the dreams reported by Dunne can be taken for granted, in a certain class of spontaneous telepathic occurrences.

However, this state of affairs is not necessarily inconsistent with the scatter theory suggested by our comparative analytical approach, nor with our insight into the structure of the unconscious mind in general. The difficulty lies elsewhere: in reconciling the current classical concepts of space and time (long discarded by contemporary physicists) with the newly established facts of psychical research. We hinted that our reference to a spatial or temporal scatter in the cases here reviewed is only due to our figurative way of speaking. We quoted Henri Bergson, the French philosopher, who went far to show that space and time in the physical sense are concepts alien to the reality of psychological processes. And we may add here that other modern philosophers are inclined to throw these obsolete categories of our thinking altogether by the board.

It is not the business of our present approach to take sides in this controversy. But whatever be its outcome, the findings of contemporary psychical research suggest that the new psychology will have to adjust its basic concepts to the fact that, apart from a few ambiguous spontaneous occurrences, we are able under special experimental conditions to catch a glimpse of a psychic reality, which, for reasons which need not be discussed at the present moment, lies beyond the range of our ordinary experience.

PART II

FRESH LIGHT ON BORDERLAND PSYCHOLOGY

Chapter V

TELEPATHY IN DREAMS*

In the first part of our inquiry we were mainly concerned with a general description of the way in which telepathy operates, with the psychological laws which it obeys, and with the method which, in our view, is best suited to the investigation of so-called spontaneous phenomena on which our chief interest is focussed in the present connection. This led to the formulation of what we termed the scatter-theory of telepathy which, we claimed, gives a fair account of the essential features of both spontaneous and experimental phenomena, not only of the ordinary, " contemporary " type but also of the still more intriguing pre-cognitive and post-cognitive types.

After these preliminaries we may feel reasonably prepared to set out for our next objective, namely, to examine a variety of problems which confront us in the field of normal and abnormal psychology in the light of the telepathy hypothesis.

The problem of telepathy in dreams may well claim the first priority in such an inquiry. The borderland between normality and mental disorder from which dreams seem to emerge, has always possessed a deep emotional appeal to mankind and thousands of years before the advent of psycho-analysis dreams have been the subject not only of man's superstitious awe, but also of his scientific curiosity. In fact the two main conflicting schools of thought regarding their origin and their meaning—which are still found in our days—can be traced back to ancient Chinese, Greek or Roman philosophers. Dreams were either considered as :

> Children of an idle brain
> Begot of nothing but vain phantasy,

or else as

> Real dreams of God,

invested with divinatory powers, with a deeper significance in

* Parts of this chapter previously appeared in the *Brit. J. Med. Psych.*, Vol. XIX, Part 2, p. 313.

which the very purpose and design of the Universe revealed itself to the sleeper. Indeed, to primitive man and to the ancients, from Homer to Plato and Cicero, the supernatural origin of dreams was beyond dispute.

But with the rationalistic trend of modern science the pendulum swung in the opposite direction. So much so, that even Freud's analytical approach to the problem, essentially rational though it has been, was originally received with a great deal of scepticism and even misgivings. To many of his contemporaries it seemed to be below the dignity of a respectable medical man to waste time with so trivial a matter as dreams, tainted with the blemish of superstitious beliefs from a bygone age. However, since the first edition of Freud's *Interpretation of Dreams*, his revolutionary theories have become almost common-place. We know now that dreams are largely derived from three sources : first, from environmental influences such as sensory stimuli, secondly, from somatic impressions, and thirdly, from the residues of past experiences which the sleeper failed duly to register or assimilate in his waking state and which, for a variety of reasons, now claim their right to be taken notice of, even at the price of disturbing his sleep.

It may be sufficient to note here in passing only that it is the third factor on which the main interest of the psychoanalytic school is centred, whilst the first two factors remain more exclusively the domain of the physiologists or psychologists moving along the beaten tracks of academic science.

However this may be, it is readily understood that there is no room left for a telepathic factor in the modern concept of dreams. It is therefore all the more remarkable that Freud himself, notwithstanding his essentially rationalistic approach, was one of the first among medical men to admit the possibility that a telepathic element may be occasionally involved in the manifest content of the dream. After having spent a life-time in building up a system of psychology from which the last trace of the irrational element has been stamped out, he thus opened up a back door, as it were, through which the old Mischief Maker could sneak in again, and there it was, much to the dislike and embarrassment of his more strictly Freudian followers.

In an essay on *Occultism and Dreams*, which first appeared in 1933, Freud discusses a dream recounted to him by the father of a married daughter who had himself married a second time and had remained childless in his second marriage. One night he dreamt that his wife had given birth to twins. The striking fact is that during the same night his daughter actually gave birth to twins, although her confinement was expected at a much later date and nobody had suspected a twin pregnancy. Freud remarks that he is not altogether convinced of the telepathic nature of the dream and that he dare not rule out the possibility of chance to account for the temporal coincidence (1) of dream and actual event, and (2) for the birth of twins reflected in the dream. Moreover, he was able to show that, whatever be the source of the manifest content of the dream, it is in good keeping with its orthodox analytical interpretation. This would suggest that the father, who is at odds with his second wife, has unconscious incest wishes towards his daughter. He would like her to take the place of his unwanted wife and this is expressed in the usual way by the dream in which it is his wife who is pregnant in his daughter's stead. But Freud points out that the psychoanalytical and the telepathic interpretation of the dream (which cannot be disregarded, after all), are by no means mutually exclusive and that the telepathic factor, so far as its existence can be taken for granted, may be subject to the same laws of distortion, condensation, secondary elaboration, etc., as other elements entering the intricate fabric of the dream.

The literature of psychical research abounds with accounts of telepathic dreams of the type described by Freud, and some of them are undoubtedly more conclusive considered as evidence for telepathy. On the other hand, they have mostly the drawback that they permit little insight into the psychological conditions on the part of the respective agent and percipient and do not therefore lend themselves to comparative analysis.

The following dream described to me by one of my patients has the advantage of an unmistakable telepathic element which can be identified in its manifest content, combined with the possibility of at least a tentative comparative analytical investigation of both agent and percipient. A school mistress of German origin, aged thirty-seven, has been under my care in a convalescent home in this country. She was suffering from nervous dyspepsia and I suspected the recrudescence of a mild cholecystitis. She was running sub-febrile temperatures for weeks and failed to respond to the usual medical treatment. I was somewhat concerned about her condition and on the night of the 10th July 1941, when again thinking over her case, I decided to try "something new". In previous years I had been advocating the method of histamine ionisation, applied to the skull, for the treatment of migraine and other vascular disorders of the brain, a procedure to which I was unable, to my great regret, to attract the attention of my British colleagues. For the sake of the non-medical reader, I may remark that histamine ionisation is a method of physiotherapy which aims at producing a local irritation of the skin, resembling a nettle-rash. Why should I not try the method in her case and carry out histamine ionisation in the region of liver and gall bladder? The erythema of the skin might entail the same beneficial effect upon the organs affected as in the case of what I called cranio-cerebral ionisation. These were my deliberations before I fell asleep.

Next morning I entered the patient's ward with my small portable ionisation apparatus: "I have something new for you, Miss N." The patient seemed apprehensive. "I hope no injections, doctor, I am so afraid. I had a strange dream. You came into this room, just as you are coming now, and I had a rash on my abdomen, a red itchy rash with small spots and weals. You looked at it gravely and then came Miss S. and said, 'Well, this is cancer, I am sure'." I asked the patient to show me the place where she had seen the rash. She pointed to her abdomen, precisely to the right hypochondric region where I was going to apply the electrodes soaked with the solution of histamine.

The patient's account of the dream was witnessed by one of her fellow patients and was repeated to the matron of the home. I may also mention that I immediately put it down in writing. The patient herself was greatly amazed by the visible local effects of the treatment. It had produced the very same spots and weals, on the same place as she had seen them in the dream, she declared. I may add here that

Miss N. had no previous knowledge whatsoever of the treatment and had not heard of it from patients on whom it had been carried out before. In this way the correspondence of the artificial nettle-rash with the motif of spots and weals in the dream, appearing precisely where the treatment was to be applied, on the very night on which I was pondering about it, is quite obvious and cannot reasonably be attributed to chance alone. The telepathic interpretation of Miss N.'s dream is therefore, to say the least, rather suggestive.

What then, are the psychological conditions for the origin of telepathy in the dream described? The part of the agent was obviously played by myself. I already hinted that I had been a fervent advocate of the method of ionisation in the past years. Indeed it would be true to say that it was one of my " emotionally coloured " pre-occupations, and at that time I was actually preparing an article on that subject. It is also true that the image of the nettle-rash, as provoked by the treatment, was not on the critical night immediately present in my mind. But it goes without saying that my preoccupation with the matter was by itself bound to evoke that image. The motif of the nettle-rash in the manifest content of the dream was in this way a typical example of telepathic scatter, as described on a previous page, resulting in the appearance of a special emotionally emphasised element from the agent's mind in the dream.

The psychological conditions on the part of the percipient are less transparent. The only factor whose significance is immediately apparent is sleep itself. We know that one of the principal characteristics of sleep is the abeyance of consciousness. In this respect sleep is a typical minus-function, as described in the previous chapter, so much so, that on the ground of our hypothesis, it should be pre-eminently suited for the origin of telepathic occurrences. But this is clearly far too general a formulation and does not account for the fact that for all we know, telepathy in dreams is the exception rather than the rule. Still less does it explain why my patient had become telepathically sensitive to an emotionally coloured idea of my own and not of somebody else, and why, of all things important to me at that time, her choice fell precisely on the proposed treatment with histamine ionisation.

Only tentative answers to these questions can be offered in the present connection. I mentioned that Miss N. had been under my care for a physical ailment and I had no opportunity of carrying out methodical psychoanalysis in her case. However, from prolonged observation it had become obvious to me that she was an anxiety neurotic with hysteric features and a pronounced masochistic attitude. This explains her aggressive interpretation of my intended treatment as reflected by Miss S.'s remark about the spots and weals which, she was afraid, might be symptoms of cancer. If this is true, my own preoccupation with the proposed ionisation treatment met half-way, as it were, her own unconscious wishes and desires with regard to my person and thus made her specifically sensitive to the matter.

On the other hand, it was mere coincidence that I happened to be right on the spot to receive the first-hand account of her dream, the hidden telepathic implications of which none but myself was in a position to appreciate. Obviously, to anybody else it would have appeared an ordinary dream with nothing to indicate its telepathic nature. It was thus the double coincidence of a special set of psychological conditions in conjunction with favourable external circumstances which accounted not only for the origin of telepathy in the dream, but also for its occurrence being realised by at least one of the persons involved.

It will be as well to note this point if we wish to arrive at a balanced picture of the part played by the telepathic factor in dreams in general. Obviously, what applies to the dream discussed here is also true for any other dream. It may or may not contain a telepathic element, but in the absence of the requisite information, which can only be derived from comparative analytical investigation of all those concerned, there is no way to find out. There is a further factor which is apt to increase the difficulties of ascertaining the telepathic nature of a certain item in the manifest content of the dream. In our case the motif of the nettle-rash was easy to identify as such an item. It had not been subjected to the distorting forces of repression, to what Freud called dream censorship. But we know that distortion, condensation, secondary elaboration, and the like, are important characteristics of the dream, especially if the item in question is in some way objectionable to the conscious self of the dreamer. Precisely the same is true for the agent. He, too, may be inclined to shut the element concerned out of his consciousness, and we have seen that this may make it particularly suitable for telepathic transmission. But at the same time his " blind spot " may render him unable to identify the item in question as " a piece of his own mind " and thus militate against its proper appreciation. To put it in other words, the telepathic factor which is woven into the fabric of a dream has to pass through the double censorship of both the agent's and the percipient's, which may in turn result in its complete assimilation by the dreamer's mind. It is readily understood that more often than not this may make the recognition of its telepathic nature very difficult indeed. On the other hand, it shows that telepathic phenomena are as a matter of principle subject to essentially the same laws as any other psychological processes that take place in the borderland between the conscious and the unconscious sphere. Indeed, we have seen that the dreamer's reaction to the foreign element intruding into his dream is precisely the same as his reaction to the intrusion of elements from his own unconscious or pre-conscious, or to such sensory stimuli as he may receive from various parts of his body during sleep. We can conveniently describe this state of affairs by saying that as a general rule, the dream may be made up of two principal parts : first, from the sum total of impressions derived from the dreamer's own conscious, pre-conscious or unconscious sphere. These we may describe as *auto-psychic* experiences. Secondly, from sources alien to the dreamer's mind, originating from another person's conscious, pre-conscious or unconscious sphere. The latter may be termed *hetero-psychic* experiences. This way of describing the part played by the telepathic element in our dream-life has obviously far reaching theoretical implications, and we shall see on a later page that it is in fact a pointer towards a deeper understanding of the role of telepathy in our mental organisation.

So far we considered only one factor which, in our view, plays an important part in the origin of the telepathic phenomena in dreams—the factor of sleep—and we paid little attention to the dreamer's personality. We have now to revert to our patient in order to examine this side of the picture. I mentioned that Miss N. had a pronounced neurotic disposition. She was of the emotionally unstable, hypersensitive type, subject to occasional hysteric fits with attacks of screaming and loss of consciousness. Her chronic dyspepsia and bilious states were obviously in part of functional origin and her history showed that they were aggravated by matrimonial difficulties. Her sex life had been abnormal from childhood. In her teens she had formed unhealthy attachments to girl friends and she had remained frigid in married life. She was never brilliant at school and later on earned her living as an uncertificated teacher. Yet, despite her limitations she was self-opinionated and liked to boast of her ability to " handle " people. She claimed that she was able intuitively to assess the personalities of her fellows. " I feel at once what kind of people I have to deal with. It is the atmosphere which I sense, whether they are good or bad, whether they like me or hate me. I get a picture of the whole person in a flash and my first impression has never deceived me." The fact is, that she sometimes showed remarkably sound judgment in this respect, whilst in other cases her diagnoses were grossly mistaken.

It is against this background that we must consider the telepathic dream just described. To this we have to add that, by her own account, it was not her only experience of this kind. In fact, she had a large stock of similar stories to tell, most of which were of a trivial nature and utterly unconvincing, adorned by colourful interpretations of her own. However, there is one story which she used to recount in a fairly consistent manner and which is of special interest in the present connection in view of its striking resemblance to many similar accounts in the literature of psychical research.

Miss N. was an only child. She lost her father early and was much attached to her step-father. In the Great War he fought on the Western Front and it was in autumn 1917 that for several weeks her family had received no news of him. On the night of the 9th August 1917—the patient was twelve years at that time—she was violently awakened from her sleep by what she thought was a terrific bang on the staircase. She woke her mother : " Mummy, something has happened to dad ! " she cried. The house was searched but nothing was found to account for the noise. A fortnight later they received a letter with the news that her step-father was killed by a shell splinter at Verdun on the night of her dream.

I am not in a position to verify this account and there is little in the mental make-up of this patient that would encourage me to take it at its face value. But the fact remains that in at least one instance her claim to be subject to telepathic or similar experiences was confirmed by direct observation and this makes the rest of her statements at least worth considering from our point of view. It suggests that, despite her grossly hysteric disposition and her tendency to indulge in day-dreams and phantasies, there may be a grain of truth in her claims and that, apart from her hysteric traits, there may be an additional feature in her mental make-up which renders her particularly prone to so-called psychic experiences. This suggestion cannot be further elaborated in the present context. It opens up the problem of the characterological aspects of telepathy which will be discussed in a later chapter. But we have to note here that a special characterological predisposition, whatever its nature, is obviously a further important conditioning factor of telepathic sensitiveness.

The dreamer of a second telepathic dream observed by myself was a highly educated lady of thirty-two, undergoing a short spell of psychological treatment. The dream goes back to her eighteenth year when she was spending her summer holidays with her parents in Carlsbad. Her father was a well-known publisher and in his company she met Mr. B., a noted painter. Mr. B. was a married man and of about her father's age. One day he suggested that he should paint a portrait of her. My patient first disliked the idea and suspected that the painter was not so much interested in herself as in the prospect of gaining publicity through her father's social connections. She was at that time intensely opposed to what she regarded as "mercenary stratagems", particularly in art and literature, an attitude she believed she had noticed in her father. Yet Mr. B. persuaded her to agree to his plan and she posed for him for a couple of weeks in his studio—it was actually rather a prosaic hotel-room—with his wife regularly present at the sittings. Mrs. B. was a beautiful woman in her thirties and she and her husband seemed quite happy together. She was polite though somewhat indifferent and my patient remarked that she disliked her condescending manner towards her.

Returning to Prague from her holidays she lost sight of the artist and his wife for several weeks. It was at that time—in September 1929—that she dreamed she came into a hotel-room where she found the painter in a state of despair, sitting in a chair. " My wife has died ", said the painter in tears. The room all around was in disorder and the dreamer felt she had come to console him and to put things right in the room. On awakening she was greatly upset by the dream. Yet she did not speak about it to anybody until the following evening when the telephone rang and she learned that Mrs. B. had died unexpectedly the night before in a Prague nursing home from a septic tooth. Now the patient revealed the dream to her relatives who confirmed to me the particulars of her account.

Here too, as in other instances of this kind, the objection of mere chance coincidence is at hand. However, it is obviously quite improbable that both the motif of Mrs. B.'s death and its temporal coincidence with the dream should have occurred in a merely fortuitous manner. The theory of gross misrecollection or even wilful misleading, though feasible by itself, is equally improbable. My patient told me the story of her telepathic dream in the course of her psychotherapy, among other things referring to her past history the veracity of which I had no reason to doubt. In fact, the dream was in good keeping with the psychological background of her case. She was suffering from an obsessional neurosis of mild degree, the detailed description of which is irrevelant to our issue. Be it sufficient to remark that it was largely due to a neurotic fixation on her father, which in later years had given way to an over-emphasised opposition to him. This was reflected in her ambivalent attitude towards the artist which made it clear that to her unconscious he was actually nothing else than a typical father representative. This was the reason for her jealousy of the artist's wife—representing the mother-image—with all its psychoanalytical implications. But if this be true the motif of Mrs. B.'s death occurring in the dream was only the familiar expression of the dreamer's repressed death wishes for her mother-image—her rival with the beloved father. This is in a nutshell, the psychoanalytical reading of the dream, and there is little doubt that, considered by itself, it offers satisfactory insight into its latent meaning.

But at the same time, it adds to our information regarding the psychological conditioning factors for the origin of telepathy on the part of the percipient. It reveals the hidden emotional significance of Mrs. B.'s death to her unconscious and makes her telepathic sensitiveness to this apparently indifferent event thus more intelligible. In other respects her dream follows the pattern of the one discussed above. Here, too, the hetero-psychic element is intimately blended with auto-psychic material which appears in the dream, although it will be noted that the salient fact—the death of Mrs. B.—has been completely spared by the distorting forces of dream-censorship. Whether this is due to the primarily strong emotional emphasis which is attached to such a dramatic event, or to the fact that it simply happened to fall within the range of what we called telepathic scatter cannot be decided in the present context. In any case, it is clear that it is especially telepathic dreams in which the hetero-psychic element is being reproduced without undue distortion which are of the greatest evidential value to the student of psychical research, and it will be recalled that failing this their telepathic interpretation may remain open to serious doubts. In fact, on sifting the evidence of telepathic dreams published in the literature, it becomes apparent that most of the "good" cases unwittingly conform with this postulate, i.e. the telepathic factor contained in the dream is readily identifiable in the manifest dream content and exhibits such distinctive features as to make chance correspondence with an actual event highly improbable.

By way of a footnote, I may quote a dream of this kind which appeared in Vol. XXVIII, p. 253, *Journ. Soc. Psych. Res.* The dreamer, Miss Mary Jones, reports as follows :

"I have to go into details to explain the circumstances ; I was on night duty (as a professional nurse) which explains why I was asleep in the day time. One evening, 18th May 1931, I was startled out of my sleep by a voice which called out my name distinctly, 'Margaret, Margaret'. I felt positive that someone had been in my room by my bed and rushed out again. I was never called by my christian name at the hospital ; however, I did not pay much attention to that as I was asleep. I thought it must have been the maid calling the night nurses and she had not switched my light on. I got out of bed and looked down the corridor, I did not hear or see anybody. I looked at my clock; it was 5.30 p.m. This was quite early as we were not called until 7.30 p.m. I sat up in bed thinking over the strangeness of the situation. However, I dropped off to sleep again.

At breakfast that night, I told some of my colleagues about my strange experience and they joked about it. I went on duty at 10.30 p.m. The night sister came to me, called me to one side, and asked me did I know anyone living at——. I said 'Yes, my sister lives there'. 'Well, nurse', she said, 'I am afraid there is bad news for you.' She handed me a telegram which said: Darling Peggy passed away at 5.30 p.m. The telegram had been opened by Sister as there were five Nurse Jones' at that particular hospital. Peggy was my little niece, aged eight years. We were great friends. She was taken suddenly ill and an immediate operation was performed, but she lived only a few hours. When I met my sister, I told her what I had experienced and she told me that the child called out 'Margaret!' and she remarked to her husband, 'Is she calling herself, or Auntie Margaret?' It is a strange fact that the stated time of the child's death on the wire was 5.30 p.m. just about the time that I was disturbed from my sleep. I did not know the child was ill; it was very sudden. I cannot describe my feelings as I read the telegram which reminded me of my strange experience at 5.30 p.m."

A corroborative statement from the child's mother is attached to this report. It reads as follows:

"This is to certify that my husband and I were present at the death of my little daughter on May 19, 1931. It is true that she called out 'Margaret' and that at the time I remarked to my husband, 'Is she calling out her own name or Auntie's?' And that two days afterwards I learned from my sister that she had been disturbed in her sleep by a voice calling out 'Margaret' (twice), and that the same evening she received a telegram from us informing her of the death of our child."

Further, one of Miss Jones' colleagues supplies the following statement:

"This is to certify I was present in May 1931 when Margaret Jones related her dream with reference to her niece calling."

This case seems to be unassailable as far as proofs are concerned, and Mr. G. N. M. Tyrrell, quoting it in his book *Science and Psychical Phenomena*, rightly remarks that it rules the theory of purposeful misreporting as well as fraud or collusion out of the question. We may, therefore, be well satisfied with the telepathic nature of Miss Jones' dream and regard it as a representative example of its kind.

It will be noted, however, that apart from furnishing a good factual report of such an occurrence it gives little insight into the psychological background of the dream. There is only one respect in which it adds to the information which we gained from the discussion of the two previous cases. It makes it highly probable that in this case the part of the agent was played by little Margaret, the dreamer's niece, in her hour of death. It is thus one of the few well attested instances of *telepathy from the dying* (such as have been reported in the literature of psychical research) and which still play a prominent part in popular belief. But if we are justified in taking occurrences of this type for granted, their value for our present inquiry is obvious. They throw light upon a new, the physiological, aspect of the origin of telepathy and show that other things being equal, physical factors affecting the function of the agent's central nerve system may play an important part in his " agency ".

Most accounts of so-called telepathy from the dying have two things in common : they are accounts of sudden or violent death of the person concerned, and they stress the emotional relationship that exists between agent and percipient. We have to comment only on the first point in the present connection.

From what we know about the physiological changes involved in the process of dying, it proceeds with a gradual dissolution first of the higher, and subsequently of the lower, centres of the central nervous system. We also know that in sudden death this may be associated with states of motor excitement, generalised convulsions or so-called decerebrated rigidity, well known from the animal experiments. We may only recall the psychological symptoms attached to partial strangulation or drowning ; the complex motor reactions observed in guillotined persons, etc. It is interesting to recall here that Hughlings Jackson, the great English neurologist, attributed reactions of this class to the sudden release of the activity of primitive strata of the central nervous system, accompanying the dissolution of the higher strata. In fact, his strata theory has gone far to explain a wide variety of symptoms, both neurological and psycholgical, along the same lines.

The relevance of this Jacksonian doctrine to our problem is obvious. It suggests that so-called telepathy from the dying can be explained in terms of Jackson's release phenomena, and it may well be that what we said on an earlier page, regarding the part played by emotional factors, psychological crises, etc., in the mental setting of the agent, may likewise be accounted for by his theory. *Mutatis mutandis*, the same may be true for what we described in such minus-states on the part of the percipient as sleep, mental dissociation or special disabilities, and their corresponding tendency to compensation. They all conform with the same pattern of neuro-physiological processes and thus once again confirm our view that, as far as the medico-psychological aspect is concerned, the phenomena discussed here are in good keeping with facts established in the field of both psychoanalysis and neuro-physiology.

Chapter VI

TELEPATHY IN THE PSYCHOANALYTIC SITUATION*

" FLECTERE si nequeo superos Acheronta movebo." † This is the motto Freud set in front of one of the earlier editions of his *Interpretation of Dreams*. My dictionary of classical quotations, giving the translation of this challenge to the Dark Powers of the unconscious, remarks, with a frown, that these are words which are only likely to proceed from the mouth of a " vindictive and unscrupulous opponent ". This judgment is, perhaps, a little harsh on Professor Freud, but there can be little doubt that he meant his challenge in earnest. He set out to purge the human mind from the last traces of the irrational element, to banish the Acherontic forces of the depths and to bring them under the undisputed sway of the conscious self. He declared that the interpretation of dreams was the Royal Road towards this objective, but the exploration of faulty actions, of obsessional habits, of the mentality of the child and of the primitive were as many avenues leading to the same goal. To-day there is wide consensus of opinion that psychoanalysis moves in the right direction, and many psychiatrists are inclined to endorse Freud's claim that he has, in point of fact, devised a method of rational psychological treatment which equals the exactness of a surgical operation or a chemical transaction.

However, it testifies to Freud's incorruptible scientific spirit that at the climax of his career he went far to revise his original uncompromising attitude towards alleged supernormal phenomena, and we pointed out on an earlier page that in so doing he threw open the gates to doubts as to the uncontestably rational nature of his system.

In the foregoing chapter I gave prominence to his account of a telepathic dream, although I had to remark that Freud

* Previously appeared in *Brit. J. Med. Psychol.*, *20* (1944).

† " If I cannot influence the gods of heaven, I will stir up Acheron itself."

himself was somewhat reluctant to accept its "supernormal" implications as an established fact. His account of further cases of telepathy in the psychoanalytic situation is qualified by similar reservations, and he openly admits having hesitated over their publication for nearly ten years "for fear of our scientific world picture being vitiated by them".

But it is clear that precise observations of this kind are of prime interest to our issue. It is true that they share most of the shortcomings intrinsic to spontaneous phenomena as far as proofs are concerned, but compared with most of the evidence presented in the literature of psychical research, observations made during the psychoanalytical situation have the great advantage that they rest on the authority of students who can claim special experience in subtle psychological observation and self-observation. Moreover, the conditions—during psychoanalysis—are for obvious reasons particularly suitable for obtaining the phenomena in *statu nascendi*, as it were, and for subjecting both the agent and the percipient to the desired comparative inquiry without delay.

We may recall Freud's first case of a lady of forty-three of whom we only learn that she was undergoing treatment for neurosis. Her analysis discovered a strong fixation on her father which prevented her finding happiness in her marriage. She was longing for children and hoped to reawaken her love for her husband by identifying him (as the father of her children) with her own father-image. When she learned there was no prospect of having children owing to her husband's illness, she became more deeply entangled in her neurosis. She was twenty-seven when she turned to a "fortune-teller" in Paris, who, taking her for unmarried, "prophesied" that she would have two children at the age of thirty-two. By the time her psychoanalysis began this prophecy had proved manifestly wrong: the patient had remained childless, and there was less hope than before of having children at the age of forty-three.

Yet her analysis showed, nevertheless, a surprising correspondence to reality with the fortune-teller's statement. The patient's mother was just thirty-two years of age when within the shortest possible interval she gave birth to two children, after almost resigning hope of having any at her age. It was clear that the patient, in her phantasy, took the place of her mother, and that the fortune-teller, by his alleged prophecy relating to an intimate detail of her mother's past life, hit upon the daughter's most ardent desire. The wish to have children—one of the implications of her father complex—governed her unconscious life for years, and its frustration was one of the precipitating factors of her illness. Thus the fortune-teller's prophecy had proved wrong, it is true, but the striking fact remains that it disclosed precisely and in fully adequate manner a distinct unconscious idea existing in the patient's mind. Since there was no conceivable means of the fortune-teller understanding the significance to the daughter of either the reference to two children or to the age of thirty-two, Freud had no option other than to attribute the incident to telepathy between the fortune-teller and his client.

We may also quote again Freud's second observation referring to a fortune-teller's prophecy. This patient, a young man, fell ill at the time of his beloved sister's wedding. In this case analysis revealed strong fixation to his sister. This did not, however, prevent him from encouraging her marriage, in spite of the disapproval of their parents. Having undergone a first series of analytic treatments the young man consulted a lady astrologer who " prophesied " her client's future by means of a horoscope starting from birth data. The young man gave her the birth data of his brother-in-law. The fortune-teller's forecast was gloomy. She prophesied that the young husband would die the next July or August from poisoning by crayfish or oysters.

Here, too, the prophecy proved entirely wrong. The brother-in-law did not die at the predicted time. Yet he had fallen ill during the past summer, before the patient had consulted the astrologer, and the cause of his illness was in fact poisoning from crayfish or oysters. Analysis made it clear that the patient had not, at that time, overcome his unconscious hatred of the rival who had married his sister. Hence his repressed wish that he might have died of the poisoning. According to Freud's conjecture he might have thought: " Such food-fads are likely to persist . . . Why should it not happen again ? " As there was no possibility of the astrologer knowing about this insignificant detail from the life history of the brother-in-law, Freud was compelled to suggest that here again this intelligence was due to some "super-normal" means of communication with the inquirer's unconscious. In this way only could the fortune-teller be supposed to have revealed to her client a certain item in his brother-in-law's biography related in a particular way to his own wishes and expectations.

We emphasised that the evidential value of these two observations is undoubtedly limited. Freud had to rely on second-hand information, and the possibility of misrecollection or misrepresentation on the part of his informants cannot entirely be ruled out. Moreover, in both cases the incident dates back some considerable time prior to its recording, viz. eleven years in the one, and several months in the other. Further, in both instances only one of the persons involved was accessible to direct inquiry, namely, the patient, whilst his or her opposite number, the fortune-teller or astrologer, remains out of the picture. It may be that it was owing to these shortcomings that Freud hesitated so long over their publication. On the other hand, he considered their evidence strong enough to justify putting forward his working hypothesis which was quoted in a previous chapter.

In a further group of observations the evidence was at least not impaired by the drawback of second-hand information. They occurred to Freud during the analytical situation, and it was he himself who seemed to be playing the role of the agent. Yet in these cases, too, Freud hesitated to acknowledge their genuineness without reservation. They are not impressive and, as so often happens in spontaneous phenomena, again are open to the objection of chance coincidence. His first observation of this type goes back to 1919, when after the Great War Freud was greatly pleased by the visit of Dr. Forsyth, the noted London analyst, to his Vienna house. Freud being engaged with a patient, Dr. Forsyth left his visiting card with the message that he would call again. While dealing with his next patient, Mr. P., Freud was still thinking of his distinguished guest—the first foreigner to visit him following the cessation of hostilities—when this patient unexpectedly produced the name *Herr von Vorsicht*. This is the German equivalent of Mr. Foresight, a name closely resembling that of Dr. Forsyth, and the patient mentioned it with reference to his own story.

From the analytical point of view this reference fits in well with the patient's general attitude to the analyst. Freud interpreted it as an expression of his jealousy of the stranger to whom the analyst's attention had been diverted from him. Here again the point is that the patient could by no conceivable " normal " means have learned of the doctor's presence in Vienna and still less of his visit to Professor Freud.

Another observation of Freud's refers to the unmotivated reference by his patient during analysis to the word " nightmare ". This occurred precisely when Freud was concerned with the presence in Vienna of another distinguished visitor from London, Dr. Ernest Jones, whose book on the *Nightmare* had aroused his keenest interest. Finally, in a third case, the name of Professor Freud's friend, *Anton von Freund*, happened to intrude into the analytical conversation in the form of the patient's slip of the tongue, just when Freud was thinking of a visit he had paid to Anton von Freund's home.

A number of similar observations have appeared in the analytical literature. Dorothy Burlingham describes a case in which mother and child were undergoing analytical treatment. One day the mother told her the story of a golden sovereign which had played a part in her childhood. On coming home from that particular session her boy, ten years of age, produced this very coin which he had picked up from among his belongings without any conceivable reason. Questioned by the analyst, the child was unable to account for his having done so. A week or so later the boy's mother was on the point of making a note of the incident when suddenly the boy turned up and demanded the sovereign. Here again, the analyst, although not fully convinced of the telepathic nature of the case, could not by any means account for the child's behaviour.

Another observation of a similar kind was reported by Helen Deutsch. One day her patient described a dream of a married couple who were celebrating the eighth anniversary of their wedding. There appeared no significant correlation between the patient's associations and this particular motif of the dream. On reflection, however, the analyst was struck to find that during the previous day's session she had been inattentive to her work owing to her preoccupation—at the back of her mind—with preparations for her own eighth wedding anniversary. It is needless to say that in this case, too, there was no reason to assume that the patient could have gathered any direct information of this intimate detail from the analyst's biography.

I. Hollós in Budapest has recorded a number of instances of what he called telepathy of everyday life, based on careful notes he had taken for many years. They refer to observations both in and outside the psychoanalytic situation and cannot here be reproduced in great detail. A number of similar observations—the original accounts of which are not accessible to the present writer—have been reported by Winterstein, Ferenczi, S. Servadio and others.*

All these instances, taken at their face value and considered by themselves, may not suffice to convince a sceptic, but their concerted evidence, in conjunction with the results of modern experimental investigations, cannot fail to carry conviction. In fact Helen Deutsch, Hollós and Servadio were satisfied with the telepathic nature of their observations and even Freud, in his latest writings, has been inclined to acknowledge their genuineness. But, strangely enough, both Freud and his followers have failed even to consider the possibility that their significance might be more than merely accidental to the psychoanalytical situation. They regard them largely as the outcome of a casual hitch in the smooth working of the treatment, due to an extrinsic disturbing factor, alien to and inconsistent with the whole psychoanalytical system of thought and the approved scheme of orthodox analytical procedure.

But as soon as we are satisfied with the factual evidence of even one of the occurrences we are confronted with a momentous question. Why, we may ask, should telepathy be confined to such insignificant happenings on the fringe of the psychoanalytic situation as we have discussed? Why should it be restricted to such comparatively trivial events as the analyst's preoccupation with preparations for a wedding anniversary or his casual inattentiveness due to the unexpected call of a foreign visitor? We have pointed out that it is the emotional

* An important contribution to the same subject by Jule Eisenbud of New York appeared since this book has gone to the press. (The Psychoanalytic Quarterly, xv. 1946).

significance to an agent's unconscious of apparently insignificant occurrences which is responsible for their becoming active in a telepathic way. This is also obviously true for the cases with which we have dealt in the present connection. But is this type of trivial thoughts and ideas the only one that is likely to gain telepathic activity in the patient's mind? Can the presence in the analyst's unconscious of elements and motifs equipped with similar (or deeper) emotional relevance to both himself and the patient be safely ruled out? Are we really to assume that such foregoing analysis as the analyst has been subjected to has succeeded in emptying out his own unconscious to the uttermost? This has, of course, never been asserted, and it goes without saying that nobody can possibly eliminate in his approach to his fellow-men a certain number of uncontrolled wishes and expectations, unformulated thoughts and ideas that might, under favourable conditions, become telepathically active.

The implications of such a suggestion are far-reaching enough. Psychoanalysis is wont to be regarded as a thoroughly rationalistic system of thoughts, based on a thoroughly rationalistic approach to the patient. Even what vestiges of primitive attempts at mental healing it originally contained—hypnosis or suggestion—are said to be eliminated from its technique, or have themselves been subjected to analytical examination. The intrusion of a telepathic factor into the psychoanalytic situation substantially alters this position. Once established, it is likely to cast doubt on the unconditionally rationalistic nature of the whole system of psychoanalysis and on the premises upon which it is based.

In fact, there is a number of features in the psychoanalytic situation which, in spite of its rationalistic design, clearly favour the origin of telepathy. There is the general rule advising the patient to assume a relaxed, passive mental attitude and to give way to any casual thought or fancy which is passing through his mind. He is called upon to divert his attention from external stimuli, to "concentrate" upon his inner experiences. Added to this is all the external make-up of his immediate surroundings, the dimmed light of the consulting room, the analyst's calm and monotonous way of speaking, the patient's recumbent position, and, last but not least, his primary neurotic mental setting which, as above stated, may itself furnish an important conditioning factor for the origin of telepathic sensitiveness.

On the other hand, we have to consider the potential activity of the analyst's own uncontrolled wishes and preconceptions of which he himself remains largely unaware. It is true, in some of the instances to which we have referred he ultimately succeeded in identifying them. But it is clear that this identification is greatly hampered as a rule by those very forces of repression or resistance which are responsible for the potential telepathic activity of the unconscious or pre-conscious material. How, then, can we expect the analyst to become aware of the very existence of such items if their telepathic activity is dependent upon their remaining below the threshold of conscious awareness? Again, how can the analyst be convinced of the potential telepathic activity of his unconscious ideas and expectations if this activity is likely to get lost whenever his conscious attention is called to them?

However, this rigid formulation of two mutually exclusive alternatives does not allow for other, intermediate, possibilities. There will always be moments when the analyst may find himself "off his guard", but when, on retrospection, he would nevertheless be able to recall what had passed through his mind. This precisely was the case in most of our examples and it may, as a general rule, occur more frequently to the novice than to the experienced *routinier*. It may account, at the same time, for the scarcity of similar reports in the published work of analytical authors of repute. On the other hand, one may expect that the approach of the enthusiastic beginner is all the more apt to be coloured by such unconscious expectations and preconceptions as might become active upon the mind of his patient. This is illustrated by a number of experiences during my own apprenticeship in the field of psychotherapy. To put them in a proper perspective it is necessary to insert a few personal remarks at this point.

Brought up in the Viennese school of psychiatry and failing to undergo systematic training analysis, I was soon equally impressed by the orthodox Freudian school of thought and by the suggestive formulations of Alfred Adler. Also, friendship with associates of Wilhelm Stekel and studies in Jung's analytical psychology led to sincere admiration of much that each in his turn had contributed to contemporary psychology. I soon realised, however, that my anxiously maintained independence, my very lack of bias towards any one of these schools, made successful work in psychotherapy rather precarious. This was particularly the case in respect of my experiences in dream interpretation. On retrospection I now see that, at certain periods, several of my patients produced dreams which seemed definitely to support orthodox Freudian views. The well-known complexes cropped up and the familiar clues for the presence of resistance, of positive or negative transference made their appearance. The patient produced the classical picture language of the unconscious as deciphered by the pioneers of dream interpretation ; an airplane was a male sex symbol, ascending a staircase an allusion to sexual intercourse, water meant childbirth and the earth a personification of the mother. The analysis worked smoothly and without a hitch ; my psychoanalytical friends were pleased with my reports although warning me at the same time of premature optimism.

They were right, as I soon realised. The short phase of initial success which often rewards the therapeutic zeal of the beginner was followed by a stand-still and this in turn by a peculiar change of course in the treatment. The patients' dreams now appeared to be coming under the sway of a new principle ; they seemed to be speaking another language, to be filled with another type of symbolic meaning. One of my patients, a married woman of thirty, was suffering from claustrophobia. In one of her first dreams she reported having stolen her father's doorkey and hidden it in her handbag. Her father was a strict and domineering type and she was brought up in constant fear of his tyrannical ways. The motifs of key and handbag seemed to have sprung straight from Freud's *Lectures on Psychoanalysis* which I had just been studying and their symbolic meaning fitted perfectly into the picture of a neurosis with an over-compensated fixation on the father and a marked castration complex.

But in the further course of treatment and after a short period of deadlock I was led to consider another reading, the " Adlerian ", which, as I distinctly remember, had at that time been looming at the back of my mind. Considered from this angle she was protesting against her feminine role, wishing to gain the upper hand over a domineering husband, a revival of the strict father. It was at that stage that she started dreaming in what might be called Adlerian terms. In one of her dreams of that period she was standing on the roof of a high building, looking down on the people in the street. The house was like the one in which she was born, but much higher. Other dreams of a similar type followed. I remember specially recording a slip of the tongue that she made at this particular time. She referred to her husband Carl as *Carola*, the feminine equivalent of his christian name, a typical faulty action on the lines of Adler's "masculine protest".

It must be admitted that these examples, however much they impressed the writer, may fail to carry conviction. It can rightly be argued that as far as the dreams are concerned their latent meaning is the same in both instances, that the discrepancy is only due to the different way of interpreting their manifest content and that the latter does not, of itself, reveal anything. These objections are undoubtedly justifiable, even when we recall that it is mainly changes in the manifest dream content, or in the vocabulary used by the dreamer, in which the telepathic influence may manifest itself. Indeed it was precisely this unmistakable change of vocabulary which caught my attention and it is on this point that our main interest centres in the present connection. However, no detailed records of the case are available at present to substantiate this impression and even if there were it would require such an elaborate exposition of all the patient's dreams and other manifestations as would be hardly justified by their merits.

It was for this reason that, while engaged in writing this chapter I was on the point of entirely dismissing the evidence of this case as unsatisfactory when a dream reported by another patient with whom I had just commenced treatment at a convalescent home in this country seemed to lend the former unexpected support. The patient, Mrs. M., a lady of twenty-eight, was suffering from anxiety neurosis, and, discussing her symptoms with a friend, I pointed out my impression that the underlying conflict in her case might prove quite superficial and easily accessible to an "Adlerian" approach. In the first session Mrs. M. stated that she never used to dream. I gave her the usual assurance that she would certainly start dreaming during the period of her psychotherapy. On the next day, in fact, she reported the following dream : " I was standing on the roof of a high building, I looked down on the people in the street . . . I held in my hand a long object, like a tube ; suddenly I dropped it and as it fell it grew longer and longer like an accordion."

The correspondence between the two dreams—the one I had recorded more than ten years previously and which I had been reconsidering from the angle of the telepathy hypothesis, and the other, dreamt by a new patient in whose treatment I was just engaged—is unmistakable. It actually is a typical instance of what is loosely termed duplicity of cases and usually ascribed to chance coincidence. Indeed, here again, it might be argued that it is largely Schilder's " uniformity of the language of the unconscious " which is responsible for the identity of the leading motifs in the two dreams. But making allowance for Schilder's argument this does not account for the far-reaching congruency of the external means, of the actual vocabulary used to express the motifs underlying both dreams. Still less does it explain the temporal coincidence of the second dream with my doubtless emotionally tinged preoccupation with the first one. This temporal coincidence, in conjunction with their similarity in substance is either inexplicable in terms of our familiar experience or is to be attributed to telepathic influences from the analyst to the patient.

Further collateral evidence in support of such a proposition appears to come from quarters whence it might be least expected : from the literature of the various schools of psychotherapy. It is true, the dogmatic follower of one or other of the schools is little likely to commit the mistake of altering, more or less deliberately, his approach to the patient. He is saved from doing so by his whole outlook and his special course of training. But the suspicion suggests itself that it is just this immunity from that kind of error which accounts for his being spared such intriguing experiences. This may also explain why no orthodox psychoanalyst appears to have ever come across patients dreaming in the " Adlerian " jargon, and why no strictly " Adlerian " analyst has observed patients using the dream codex of the orthodox psychoanalyst, to say nothing of the prodigious mythological dreams produced by patients studied by the Zürich school.

But the problem, formulated in this way, may well tend to over-stress the discrepancies of the rival schools. One might argue that practically any dreamer is liable to dream "both ways"; that, in point of fact, it is only the manifest dream content that is found at variance and that it is a matter of interpretation how far we claim to find a latent meaning of this type or that behind the manifest dream content. But we have emphasised that it is precisely this discrepancy in the superficial aspect of dreams which has to be accounted for. When studying the dreams recorded by the Analytical or Individual psychologist or Zürich school, we cannot help feeling confronted with completely divergent styles in the self-expression of the unconscious. "Adlerian" patients seem never to be "eclectic". They appear to be persistently dreaming in their special fashion; so likewise are the patients of many orthodox analysts and of a few dissenters among them. They seem to be assiduously moving along their allotted tracks without a chance of slipping into another, simply owing to the firm and undivided attitude of their respective analysts.

This is not less striking in the contributions of the Zürich school. Jung's patients, at certain periods of his work, furnished ample evidence of uncommon abilities and hyper-functions peculiar to the unconscious. At a later period the dreams of his patients were full of grandiose allusions to the early history of our race, containing sometimes literal translations of ancient Egyptian, Assyrian and Hindu myths.

A striking example of a telepathic leakage in the psycho-analytic situation is represented by Dr. John Layard's account of his analysis of the dreams of the patient described by him as the Lady of the Hare. This patient seems to confirm all the claims of analytic psychology and in particular all the theories held by the author of the book. Certainly no reader of Layard's *Lady of the Hare* will deny the inner consistency of his interpretations. They undoubtedly "make sense" both to the analyst and his patient. But the reader will also note that no one but Layard himself could have possibly arrived at such an ingenious reading of his case. The reason is obvious : the dreams dreamt by the Lady of the Hare are the joint product of the patient's and the analyst's unconscious. Layard has been the author not only of the book, but also of a considerable part of the material upon which it is based. This is why he, and he alone, holds the key to the puzzle contained in the dreams described.

Other followers of Jung's have afforded very impressive observations of the same kind. In their cases likewise, the question arises whether a possible telepathic activity of unconscious memories of their own elaborate reading in mythology and archaeology can be safely ruled out. Jung himself has considered such a possible objection. He felt satisfied with the absence of anything like cryptomnesia on his part which would permit the origin of telepathy. But there is undoubtedly a potential source of error which must be taken into serious consideration in any further discussion not only of the interpretations of the Zürich school, but of the conflicting readings which are offered by the protagonists of psychological sects of all denominations. They may all be right when they feel satisfied with the authenticity of their claims, they may all be certain they are reporting nothing but facts of their daily experience. But there is another fact that cannot possibly be explained away: the striking contradictions of their observations, notwithstanding their indisputable individual reliability. Telepathy from analyst to patient, unaccounted for to all intents and purposes, but all the more to be suspected, may give the key to this puzzle. It may explain the inconsistencies of the findings presented by various students, in the same way as it may account for some of the present writer's own intriguing experiences at the time of his wavering at the cross-roads between the rival schools.

Similar considerations must be borne in mind with regard to other productions of the patient during the analytical situation. We have learnt from Freud that most of the patient's neurotic symptoms, his free associations, his faulty actions, his transference, his whole attitude towards the analyst obey essentially the same laws as his dreams. It would be tempting to inquire if and to what extent in these manifestations telepathic influences from the analyst can likewise be detected. But only a few passing references may be ventured in this direction. Here again, the first thing to strike us is the unmistakable variance of certain aspects of symptomatology and of case histories as presented by the various schools. There seems to be a marked difference between " first recollections " or " early memories " as elicited by each of them. Sexual traumata seem to prevail in the one whilst the struggle for self-assertion would appear to be the patient's exclusive concern in the other. A special attachment of the patient to the analyst, the so-called transference, is considered the basis of psychoanalytical treatment by the psychoanalysts, whilst Adler and his disciples bluntly deny its existence. The same considerations are true for the bewildering contradictions of the various schools of child psychology.

These divergencies are still more striking if we extend our inquiries into the past. Mesmer firmly believed in the evidence of what he called animal magnetism and he never failed to demonstrate in his sittings with his patients the most spectacular proofs of its existence. Dr. Braid of Manchester, who made history through his researches in hypnotic phenomena, was convinced of the existence of so-called phreno-magnetic points on the head, pressure on which was supposed to lead to the manifestation of various " idealities " such as veneration, self-esteem, benevolence, etc. As a matter of fact, he succeeded in demonstrating such responses in hypnotised subjects, thus confirming contemporary ideas of phrenology. Again, Charcot's hysterics seem to have specialised in producing fits of the type of the *grande hystérie* strictly in keeping with the theories of the Wizard of the *Salpêtrière*. We are now wont to hold that both the symptoms induced and the cures effected were largely due to suggestion and hypnosis. But it must remain a matter for further investigation whether or not in the classical conception of hypnosis and suggestion itself a telepathic factor is involved.

So far we have only considered instances of assumed telepathy from the analyst to the patient. Is there, one may ask, any evidence of influences in the reverse direction, that is, from the patient to the analyst? The fact is, that no first-hand observation of this kind is contained in the material here reviewed. This is readily understood if we realise one of the difficulties inherent in the method of comparative analysis of both agent and percipient as here adopted, implying as it does a combination of the roles of reliable observer (and self-observer) and successful percipient. However this may be, it does not, nevertheless, appear accidental that the acknowledged rules of psychoanalytical technique demand from the analyst a mode of procedure which, stripped of its accessories, closely resembles the mental attitude which we found to be one of the main prerequisites of telepathic sensitiveness.

Freud advises the adept to " yield himself passively to the patient's unconscious ". He is expected to meet him in a state of " suspended attention ", to dispense with seeking to grasp his problem in a merely intellectual way. Edward Glover, in his outline of the technique of psychoanalysis, has fully adopted these recommendations. Ferenczi urged the analyst to give " full indulgence to his unconscious " whilst Richard Sterba emphasised the importance of " mental relaxation ", of complete " freedom from inner tension " on his part. In short, there is much in common in the methods by which psychotherapist and telepathic percipient render their minds " blank " and susceptible to influences from each other. This gains added significance if we recall that in certain neurotics the patient's repressed unconscious tendencies may themselves assume telepathic activity. This, for instance was the case in Freud's two patients to whom we have referred. So much so, that his hypothesis of telepathy actually took shape from such observations.

But on reviewing my own records over a period of more than ten years, I must admit my inability to find a single case in which telepathy from the patient to the analyst could be detected with a reasonable degree of certainty. There are a number of instances which are very suggestive and many students may have gained similar impressions, but here, again, the available evidence is open to various interpretations and a telepathic reading is never conclusive. Obviously it is this ambiguous character of a part of the analyst's insight into an understanding of his patient's mind that gave rise to the theory of intuition as an important factor in psychoanalysis.

This is not the place to discuss the widely conflicting views held on this new element which enters the scene of the psycho-analytic situation. But there is little doubt that ultimately this factor, too, will be found to contain a marked telepathic element. It is true that Freud himself hardly attributed more significance to the problem of intuition than to telepathy itself. There is obviously no room for this essentially non-rational item in his strictly rationalistic system. In the writings of his followers, also, intuition remains only a side-issue and no serious attempt has yet been made at its reconciliation with the main teachings of psychoanalysis. On the other hand, we see that C. G. Jung and Dr. H. G. Baynes in this country, who made far-reaching allowances as to the role of intuition in psychotherapy, have finally broken away from the orthodox school, whilst Hans Prinzhorn, who put intuition right in the centre of his system—with definite leanings to the philosophies of Ludwig Klages and Henri Bergson—completely emancipated himself from Freud's original teachings.

It is readily understood why the part allotted by orthodox analysts to telepathy in the psychoanalytic situation can be after all only that of a casual and accidental side-effect. Whatever further allowance they would make for an essentially non-rational and uncontrollable factor is bound to effect the very foundation of a system which from the outset was bent on eliminating root and branch that very element from its theoretical and therapeutical equipment. But does this mean that this intrinsic aversion is really justified ? Does it indicate that the intrusion of the telepathic factor is bound to upset—if not to nullify—some of the fundamental propositions of contemporary deep psychology ?

There is a further aspect of our problem which we have failed to appreciate so far and which must be taken into account when trying to answer this question. Whatever a critical revision of the case of psychoanalysis from the angle of the telepathy hypothesis may reveal, it must be realised that only part of the fundamental principles of Freud's doctrine was arrived at in the actual situation of psychological treatment. A considerable portion is derived from sources in which bias due to emotionally coloured preconceptions—and their potential telepathic leakage—are clearly ruled out of the question. We may recall the wealth of recorded material, of biographic and autobiographic accounts and diaries which have successfully been subjected to psychoanalytical interpretation, with results identical to those arrived at through personal contact between analyst and analysand. To this may be added the evidence afforded by all the works of art, of poetry and of fiction that were subjected to the same method ; the artistic productions of primitive man, his myths, legends and fairy tales. Freud's analysis of the Oedipus drama, Rank's reading of the myth of the birth of the hero, Ernest Jones' interpretation of Shakespeare's Hamlet have become so many corner-stones in the structure of psychoanalysis being unaffected by such objections as can rightly be raised in view of the evidence for telepathy in the psychoanalytic situation.

The same refers to what the analytical appreciation of the schizophrenic psychoses has brought to light. In these instances the unconscious is laid bare to direct inspection, as it were, and the findings of Bleuler, Jung, Baynes and other investigators resulted, in spite of divergencies, in further corroboration of Freud's original concepts.

In fact, it will be noted that notwithstanding the reluctance of the orthodox analytical approach to acknowledge the existence of telepathy, our argument has itself been largely based on certain essential presuppositions of psychoanalysis. We shall see in the sequel that a proper appreciation of the telepathic factor will actually help further to deepen and extend the insight gained by the modern schools of " deep " psychology.

Chapter VII

TELEPATHY AND MEDIUMISTIC TRANCE

In the introductory chapter of this book, I explained that contemporary spiritualism is like a mountain peak of a submerged prehistoric continent projecting into the world of to-day: a strange sample of ancient primitive mentality. Modern spiritualism still maintains the belief in personal survival after death, in thought and action at a distance, and in the possibility of mind acting directly upon matter. The present context is not concerned with an inquiry into the curious collection of manifestations, mental and physical, which is put on show in the spiritualistic seance room for appropriate fees, but there is one peculiar condition upon which the majority of the phenomena hinges and which is of special interest from the angle of the telepathy hypothesis: the conditions of mediumistic trance.

What is mediumistic trance?

Its psychiatric interpretation is obvious. It is a state of mental dissociation, hysteric in origin, induced by suggestion or auto-suggestion in persons with a particular tendency to give way to such influences. The trance state, once established as an habitual pattern of reaction, gives the person concerned an outlet for unconscious or repressed tendencies which are prevented from being expressed in ordinary life. The productions of the mediumistic trance are in this way largely comparable with the familiar symptoms of hysteria and especially of hysteric multiple personality. C. G. Jung, in one of his early writings, gave a detailed analysis of such a case.

The patient was a young girl aged fifteen, of poor parentage. In the trance state she used to produce a number of imaginary personalities whose demeanour and way of speaking she assumed, and indeed, whose part she played with all the dramatic detail of a genuine stage production. One of her impersonations was the medieval knight *Ulrich von Grebenstein.* Jung was able to show that this figure was nothing else than the projection of one of her own complexes into the outer world, of part of her own self, longing for gallant deeds, heroic adventure, masculine self-assertion. Another of her trance personalities was the romantic *Lady Ivenes.* According to Jung, the creation of this figure was inspired by the patient's passionate reading of Justinus Kerner's book about the *Seeress of Prevorst* who was herself something like a trance medium in the guise of eighteenth-century romanticism.

Such accounts of mediumistic trance as are found in the spiritualistic literature tell much the same story, although in different words. They are largely determined by the preconceived ideas and theories held in the various spiritualistic sects, especially the so-called survival-hypothesis, the hypothesis of direct or indirect spirit control, etc. But stripped of these accessories the psychological pattern of mental dissociation and the production of secondary personalities derived from the medium's unconscious is easily discernible. In many cases of this type, the medium is in the habit of impersonating a fictitious personality bearing some high-sounding or exotic name, pretending to be the re-incarnation of some famous personage of a past age, of a legendary figure, or of some other deceased person who, for one reason or another, possesses a special emotional appeal to the medium or her "sitters". The utterances made by these trance personalities are then attributed to the spirits of the dead and described as spirit messages derived from so-called communicator personalities.

For instance, shortly after the death of Frederic Myers, a founder of the Society for Psychical Research, it was claimed that his spirit communicator appeared in the trance of Mrs. Piper, a well-known medium, through whom he tried to resume contact with his friends and associates. The accounts relating such phenomena follow a stereotyped pattern. Thus reports of the Piper trance simply refer to Myers_{P}, adding the medium's initial as a modest suffix only to his name in order to imply tacitly that his personal appearance was, in fact, a foregone conclusion. In the same vein, Mrs. Willett—Lord Balfour's favourite medium—was in the habit of producing the spirit of Edward Gurney, Frederic Myers' collaborator, as her regular visitor from the " unseen world ". He was then simply referred to as $Gurney_W$.

It is difficult to disentangle facts from fancies in such highly coloured reports. Some of them undoubtedly make a genuine attempt to give an honest account of the medium's behaviour and often rather rambling soliloquies in the trance state. A typical example of this kind is the description by Miss Radclyffe Hall and Una Lady Troubridge, of their sittings with the medium Mrs. Osborne Leonard, published in 1917 in the *Proceedings* S.P.R. G. N. M. Tyrrell, in his book entitled *Science and Psychical Phenomena*, testifies to their *bona fides* and actually chose theirs as a model of an investigation conducted with " an admirable care and scientific caution ". On the recommendation of Sir Oliver Lodge, the sitters consulted the medium anonymously in order to forestall any possible attempt on her part to gather information regarding their personal circumstances. They went even so far as to employ a private detective to find out if Mrs. Leonard had tried to make inquiries by some devious means, although, on Mr. Tyrrell's view, this suspicion was groundless from the outset. He emphasises the excellent reputation Mrs. Leonard enjoyed " for considerable caution and for the desire to assist the scientific precautions taken by the investigators ".

The seances were held with only two sitters present. Various trance-communicators purported to appear, among them *Feda*, an Indian girl, one of the stock characters of Mrs. Leonard's trance. However, the main interest of the seance was focussed on the appearance of a certain Mrs. A. V. B., an intimate friend of Miss Radclyffe Hall with whom she was living for some time prior to the sittings. Mrs. A. V. B. was an elderly lady who had died on the 25th May 1916, following an apoplectic seizure. In a seance on 16th August 1916, Mrs. Leonard describes the presence of an elderly lady : " The lady is of medium height, has rather a good figure but is inclined to be too fat . . . she has a straight nose, a well shaped face . . . the eyebrows are slightly arched ; the hair is not done professionally ".

One of the sitters asks : " Is it worn on the neck ? "

" No, it is done on the crown of the head. She has passed over just recently. She has not been well for some time prior to passing. . . . You were much with her in her life, you gave her vitality."

The author's remark on this statement: "A. V. B. was fifty-seven when she died, had a fine figure but latterly became too stout; she had a straight nose . . . she wore her hair dressed high on her head and at the time of these sittings she had only been dead for two months, three weeks and a day. For some time prior to her death, she had not been strong . . . A. V. B. and I were the closest of friends for eight years . . . She would sometimes say to me that my vitality kept her up and helped her; we used to discuss that together."

Miss Radclyffe Hall and her friend had been much devoted to a place at Teneriffa, Barranca Avingo, a rocky valley transversed by a lava road. In one of the sittings, Mrs. Leonard described "this very place", rock strewn, with scorching sunshine and a road where she felt like walking on cinders.

The sitters remark on this passage: "That is precisely what the road is composed of". The medium described the place as an island but had apparently great difficulties in getting its name. "The place is called Ter- Ter- Terra- Oh! Feda can't get it, but it starts Ter. It's Tenr- Tenr-, etc."

These samples from a very rich material may suffice for our purpose. They show in an instructive manner that if we strip the account of the situation from its external make-up, the gist of a simple telepathic experiment remains with the familiar tendency to telepathic scatter, to "tap" the unconscious or pre-conscious of the sitters and to produce a jumbled medley of its contents. In short, if there is a nucleus of genuine phenomena in the trance manifestations described here it is constituted by "telepathy between the living" and has nothing to do with spirit messages from the dead.

In point of fact, what we learn about the mental setting on the part of both the medium and the sitters is in good keeping with the telepathy hypothesis. The medium is in a state of pronounced mental dissociation, with her consciousness clouded or completely in abeyance. This represents what we described as a minus function on the part of the percipient and regarded as one of the principal prerequisites of telepathic sensitiveness. However, by contrast to most examples of telepathy reviewed so far, we must assume that in this case the minus function is not confined to a narrow range of cognitive processes. It embraces the whole range of consciousness, comparable to conditions of hypnosis and of hysteric fugues. If we recall our thesis of the tendency to compensation for an existing minus function, such conditions would well account for the remarkable extent of sensitiveness to hetero-psychic material which may be attained in the trance state.

Again, the role of the sitters is obviously one of the involuntary agents in a telepathic experiment and, for this very reason, particularly suitable for this purpose. On their own admission the declared aim of the sitters in the A. V. B. case was a scientific inquiry into trance-mediumship. They did not intend to play anything like the part of telepathic agents. But this precisely is one of the reasons why the experiment worked so well. To this comes that, despite the ostensibly detached scientific approach which they assumed, they undoubtedly embarked upon their inquiry with the expectation that something out-of-the-way was going to happen. Miss Radclyffe Hall stresses her affectionate friendship with Mrs. A. V. B. Indeed, her account of the experiments makes the strong emotional significance to her of all the minute recollections of the departed friend obvious; and this is, for all we know, an important factor in favour of a person becoming a successful agent. Another factor which may work in the same direction lies in the fact that, more often than not, the attention of the sitters will be diverted from what is really going on in the trance situation. It will be focussed on the expectation that supernatural things are going to take place, that spirits from another world are going to appear and that communication between those present and their departed dear ones will be established. This is precisely the right frame of mind for the origin of the phenomena.

What then, one may ask, is the difference between such cases of mediumistic trance as were described by C. G. Jung, and the trance-mediumship of Mrs. Osborne Leonard?

An orthodox spiritualist would describe Jung's observation as a case of fictitious or spurious trance-manifestations, produced by a bad medium, by contrast to the Leonard-trance which he would regard as the production of a first-class medium, with a high degree of *prima facie* evidence of "supernormality". From the medico-psychological point of view there is no fundamental difference between the two instances. In both cases secondary personalities emerged during a state of mental dissociation, following the familiar pattern of multiple personalities in hysteria. But there is one distinction which we have to point out here. Jung has shown that the trance-personalities of his patient were exclusively derived from her own unconscious wishes and desires, from what in an earlier chapter I described as auto-psychic material. By contrast, from what we have learned of the Leonard-trance there is ample evidence of a telepathic factor being involved in her productions, that is to say, we have to assume that they were in part derived from hetero-psychic sources: from material originating in the pre-conscious mental content of the sitters.

It will be noted that the way in which this hetero-psychic material makes its appearance in the trance closely resembles the manner in which hetero-psychic elements may be woven into the intricate fabric of the dream. Indeed, the psychological mechanism is largely the same in the two cases. We emphasised that in many instances it may be difficult to identify the hetero-psychic origin of the element concerned owing to the operation of dream-censorship. The same is true for the mediumistic trance. Here, too, secondary elaboration, condensation and other distorting factors may cause only fragments of the telepathic message to come "through". The medium may be side-tracked from the essential to the accidental; she may slip from the real thing to its symbolic representation; her responses may be scattered around the agent's central idea in the perspective of both time and space. This would then account for both the peculiar, vague and ill-defined nature of many trance communications and—occasionally—even for post-cognitive or pre-cognitive reactions which may in turn give rise to various misinterpretations. However, it may be found that a greater part of the usual trance productions consists of auto-psychic material only which possess all the characteristic features of the dream. Again, in other cases, it may be difficult to separate the auto-psychic from the hetero-psychic element without a thorough comparative analysis.

This explains why even confirmed spiritualists may have to admit that on closer scrutiny the majority of mediums produce spurious or fictitious trance communicators only, that is to say, multiple personalities, derived from autopsychic material, and therefore of purely hysteric origin, as was the case with Jung's patient and her romantic knight Ulrich von Grebenstein or her Lady Ivenes.

So much about the medium's contribution to the picture of mental trance phenomena. We have now to consider the part played by the presumable agents in the experiment. We cannot hope to receive much assistance in this respect from the average sitter in a spiritualistic séance. In contrast to the psychoanalytical situation, conditions in the séance room are hardly compatible with an attitude of sober psychological observation and self-observation. But from what we can read between the lines of the usual reports, it is obvious that precisely the tense, emotional atmosphere—so characteristic of the sittings—may be an ideal condition for the production of the expected phenomena. To this we have to add the dimmed light of the séance room, the monotonous background music provided by specially selected gramophone records and by prayers or hymn singing. If, in addition to this external make-up, one or the other of the sitters happens to be bereaved of one of his dear ones, pondering over his loss and preoccupied with his recollections of the departed, he will eagerly acknowledge the slightest sign purporting to indicate his presence, and the scene will be set in an ideal manner for whatever show the entranced medium may produce. Little wonder that in these circumstances the trance may work like a magic mirror, as it were, reflecting the lingering hopes and forlorn memories of those looking into it. The startling effect of such an optical illusion may be reinforced if the agent concerned fails to realise that one or the other of the items brought out by the medium is actually part and parcel of his own pre-conscious or unconscious mind.

The spiritualistic trance is in this way an experiment with telepathy, conceived on erroneous lines and conducted under thoroughly objectionable conditions, but resulting in the emergence of phenomena which throw significant light upon the psychological factors involved. In fact, it is a model case of what on an earlier page I described as para-experimental telepathy and I emphasised that the part played by this factor cannot possibly be over-estimated in psychological investigations in general. It may falsify the results not only of experiments with freely chosen material but also of card-calling tests under otherwise fool-proof conditions. We have seen in the foregoing chapter that it may even influence the course of psychotherapy and determine the pattern of dreams produced in the psycho-analytical situation in accordance with unconscious wishes and expectations of the respective analysts.

But whilst the psychotherapist is at pains to put a brake on the irrational forces which may be operative at the back of his mind, or to make them at least subservient to the aim of his treatment, they remain utterly unchecked in the spiritualist séance room. Indeed, both the medium and the sitters are at complete liberty to indulge in their collective wish dreams and phantasies, canalised, as it were, by the traditional spiritualist faith. This is why a "good" medium may have no difficulty in furnishing evidence of whatever her sitter is desirous to prove: here, as in other walks of life, the "customer" is always right. Some hundred and fifty years ago it was Mesmer's doctrine of animal magnetism in whose favour evidence seemed to be forthcoming; fifty years later it was Justinus Kerner's theory of the Sun-Sphere and its mystic relation with the Life-Sphere, or what not, and we hinted that much in the same way Charcot's concepts of *la grande hysterie* may have been tinged by unconscious telepathic leakage from the *Wizard of the Salpêtrière* on to his patients.

A striking account of what has obviously been due to similar influences from the experimenter upon his subject is contained in Lord Balfour's description of his sittings with Mrs. Willett, his favourite medium. Some of Mrs. Willett's trance manifestations seem to represent a class of their own. Among other things she was subject to what Lord Balfour described as autonomous trance, that is to say, of a trance without the appearance of the usual trance communicators or trance personalities. In these states she purported to establish direct communication with the "spirit world". Her demeanour in these states would vary between the attitude of an enchanted spectator enjoying visions of transcendental beauty but struggling with the difficulty of expressing in human language what she saw, and the cryptic utterances of a person who is herself involved in events taking place in a sphere beyond Space and Time. One of these scenes she describes as follows :

> " It is a picture that I loved and had often seen. Marble pillars everywhere—a most heavenly scene. A company of men, small company, discussing everything on heaven and earth, and really reaching the heights of reason—almost unconscious of their visible surroundings. It is a sort of parable life. There was such an intercourse of human mind going on in that room, and I know it so well I almost fancy I must have been there, though it happened a long time ago. . . . There is a poem of Matthew Arnold's about Christ, that whenever the feet of mercy move up and down where poverty is, Christ is actually present in them now. . . . Oh, how I wish I could tell you what I know. You know, to ordinary people those men who sat talking there long ago are just historical figures, interesting from a hundred points of view, but dead men. Do you know there is nothing dead in greatness. . . . I live with especially the older men, the Master. He has disciples, you know. What I said about Matthew Arnold's poem was because I wanted to say that what was true of Christ is true of the man I am speaking about. . . ."

Lord Balfour, the philosopher and statesman, assuring the reader " that Mrs. Willett's education certainly did not provide her with the chance to acquire anything that can be called even elementary classical knowledge ", intimates that in his view her account bears striking resemblance to the scenes described in Plato's *Symposion.* From this and a variety of similar observations he concludes that her productions were in fact based on information gained in some " supernormal fashion ".

From our point of view, productions like these are only fresh evidence of para-experimental telepathy, testifying to the remarkable range of sensitiveness to hetero-psychic material which may be attained during the trance states. It certainly far surpasses what telepathy in its original meaning could possibly be expected to do and there is undoubtedly a far cry from the concept of a transmission of isolated sense data, of " thought-reading " or " thought-transference " to Mrs. Willett's awareness of hetero-psychic material in the wider sense during the trance state.

On another occasion, Mrs. Willett gave an account of what in common parlance would be described as the apparition of a spirit : " I was sitting idly . . . when I became aware so suddenly and strangely of Frederic W. H. Myers' presence that I said 'Oh!' as if I had run into someone unexpectedly. During what followed I was absolutely normal. I heard nothing with my ears, but the words came from outside into my mind as they do when one is reading a book. . . ." In a ductus of automatic writing she reproduced ostensibly direct utterances of her spirit visitor: "I am trying experiments with you, to make you hear without writing. Therefore it is I, Myers, who do this deliberately, do not fear or wince when words enter your consciousness, or subsequently when words are in the script, do not analyse whence these impressions . . . come from, they are parts of a psychic education, framed by me for you. . . ." In a similar vein she reproduced whole passages of posthumous utterances, purporting to originate from E. Gurney: "Oh, he says, telepathy's one thing—that's thought communication, telesthesia is a bedrock truth, a power of acquiring knowledge direct without the intervention of the discarnate mind. . . . Oh, he says, telepathy's one thing—that's thought communication; telesthesia is knowledge, not thought . . . etc."

Seen from the angle of the psychiatrist such an account can hardly fail to be ascribed to hallucinations, strongly suggestive of hysteric origin. But here again, as in the case of trance personalities, there is one point of difference. Hallucinations of this kind may contain elements derived from hetero-psychic sources *in addition* to auto-psychic material. They may then assume the appearance of such a degree of life-like authenticity as to give rise to exaggerated claims and misrepresentations even by intelligent observers. Indeed, the striking individual quality of some of these manifestations has led to a great deal of scholarly controversy in authoritative quarters of modern psychical research. In the view of Kenneth Richmond, editor of the Journal S.P.R., the "characteristic drive and manner of self-expression of certain trance communicators so much resembles real personality as to make them difficult to explain in terms of the telepathy hypothesis alone". He admits that this may be largely due to a dramatic elaboration of the telepathically received material and reinforced by an "automatically organised system of safe guesses" but he is inclined to seek at least part of the sources of trance manifestations of this kind in some psychic entity, located outside the mental range of either the medium or the sitters.

This view is largely inspired by Dr. C. D. Broad's famous compound hypothesis. Professor Broad suggests that the living organism is a compound of an organic and a psychic factor, just as a chemical compound may be constituted by two elements. Death entails the dissolution of this compound with the destruction of the organic component, yet with the survival of the psychic factor. This may be only temporarily united with the organism of the entranced medium and thus account for the short-lived appearance of genuine trance personalities.

However, K. Richmond, G. N. M. Tyrrell and others have rightly called attention to the close similarity of the creation of trance personalities and the impersonation of stage characters by a good actor. These impersonations, too, may attain a remarkably high degree of integration, hardly inferior to the authenticity of alleged trance personalities. But instead of deriving his material from hetero-psychic sources, like a genuine medium, or impersonating some unconscious undercurrent of his own mind, like the hysteric, the actor takes his cues from his script and projects the day-dreams of Sophocles, or Shakespeare, or of Shaw, as the case may be, on to the stage. The creation of trance personalities is in this way a counterpart of the artist's creative activity and it may well be that at bottom it is of the same order as the creative imagination which is at work in our sympathetic understanding of the implicit motives of our fellows, of their likes and dislikes, of their moods and idiosyncrasies from minute clues, sensory and extra-sensory. How far the instinctive adjustment of the child to his parents and educators, his ability to learn and to receive a rounded picture of a highly complex situation from scraps of information, is based on the same principle must be a matter for further investigation.

It will be noted that all these instances have one thing in common: the remarkable tendency of integration of more or less isolated elements into organised wholes. This is in fact a basic property not only of the human mind but of life in general in both its organic and psychological aspects. The Lord God took a rib from Adam while he was asleep and so made Eve his wife. This parable expresses a principle well known to biology. We have learned from the experimental zoologist that specks of protoplasm taken from a fertilised egg cell of lower animals are capable of developing into organised wholes (into multiple personalties, as it were) in much the same way as the original germ cell. In a similar fashion a good trance medium may integrate scraps of hetero-psychic material, derived from another person's mind, into highly organised wholes, with all the attributes of "autonomous psychic entities". The emergence of trance personalities through the coalescence of a few casual hetero-psychic clues is thus comparable with the autonomous growth and tendency to self-completion of a living graft transplanted from one mind to another. Dropping the simile, it is safe to say that in any case, the basic facts established by modern configuration psychology give a more plausible account of certain intriguing aspects of the trance state than the survival hypothesis.

To sum up, trance personalities may be exclusively derived from what we called auto-psychic material. They are then described as fictitious, or spurious trance personalities, and must be regarded as nothing else than dramatic impersonations of the medium's own repressed tendencies, day-dreams and phantasies. Alternatively, they may be due to the elaboration and dramatic impersonation of hetero-psychic influences derived from unconscious or pre-conscious day-dreams and phantasies or other mental content of the sitters. We have seen that an essentially identical mechanism may be operative in the dream, although it is true to say that owing to the special characterological disposition of trance mediums, trance itself may be a much more fertile breeding ground of telepathic phenomena than ordinary sleep.

Little more can be said at the present stage of our inquiry about the characterological aspects of trance mediumship, except one thing: it bears unmistakable resemblance to such hysteric features as the tendency to mental dissociation and easy suggestibility. But to this we have to add two qualifications. First, telepathy and related phenomena are obviously not confined to the hysteric character. Indeed, they seem to be more particularly the prerogative of a characterological type of its own which may be described as the psychic type, closely related to, but not identical with, the hysteric type of character. This is in fact best illustrated by the example of the trance mediums discussed here. But to this we have to add that if hysterics are easily suggestible, prone to mental dissociation and indulgence in day-dreams and phantasies, such trance mediums as we have just described seem to be equally able to draw on hetero-psychic sources to this end, to adopt the day-dreams and phantasies of other persons in a telepathic way, and to indulge in them as if they were of their own making. Dubious though the gratification may be which can be derived from this psychic parasitism, as it were, it is perhaps the only real reward such mediums reap for their self-display to the public.*

* In fairness to the views held by many students of psychical research it must be admitted that such evidence as has been adduced in so-called proxy-sittings, and cross correspondences, etc., cannot easily be accounted for by the telepathy-hypothesis alone. More recently the question has been reviewed by Dr. Gardner Murphy in a series of important articles in the *Journal* of the American Society for Psychical Research.

PART III

FRESH LIGHT ON PSYCHIATRY

Chapter VIII

TELEPATHY AND PARANOIA

In the foregoing chapter I described a group of eccentric personalities in whom certain hysteric features of character are coupled with a predisposition to telepathic and related experiences. I stated that persons of this "psychic" type may indulge in, and derive gratification from, day-dreams and phantasies which intrude into their consciousness from deeper strata not only of their own minds, but also from the minds of other persons. They are suggestible both in an "ordinary" and in an "extraordinary" way, whatever the term may be taken to indicate. This type of character seems to be in striking contrast to the so-called paranoic or schizophrenic reaction type as described by clinical psychiatry.

In the following chapters I propose to show, first, that patients suffering from paranoia in a stricter sense, or from paranoic schizophrenia at the initial stages of the process, respond to the same things in precisely the opposite manner; second, that this reaction may play an important part in the gradual disintegration of the personality in the further course of the process. I will try to sum up the information gained from this new, and admittedly, unorthodox approach to the problem of schizophrenia in Chapter X, dealing with the clinical picture of the disorder as seen in the light of the telepathy hypothesis.

Attacking one of the major problems of contemporary psychiatry from this angle is treading on treacherous ground; and is, in any case, in need of vindication. Objection may be raised that an attempt at a telepathic interpretation of the paranoic reaction type bears a suspicious resemblance to the patient's own reading of his case. So common is, indeed, the allegation by the patient that he is being subjected to telepathic or mediumistic influences, or that he himself possesses supernatural powers of thought or action, that the psychiatrist will always regard with suspicion the very sanity of a person putting forward such claims. He knows that ideas of this kind are well-nigh symptomatic of mental disease and that the majority of future schizophrenic patients is likely to pass through a paranoic phase. In many cases the patient's statements, which are suspicious in this respect, may be vague and confused, lacking consistency and elaboration. In others, they may be woven into a coherent pattern of systematised delusions of persecution or grandeur, barely distinguishable from the theories which are presented by the advocates of the " occult ". This is especially true of the so-called spiritualistic psychoses in which popular fallacies and superstitions imperceptibly merge into what appears a survival from the magic and animistic world outlook of primitive man.

One of my patients, a woman of average education, evolved an elaborate system of this type. I quote the following passage from a lengthy poem :

" Fear is the most unpleasant sensation,
That upsets the Psychic vibrations,
Some people have this evil power,
And throw it off in a vicious hour.
There is no need for physical connection,
When the victim takes this condition.
It is a case of thought-transmissions,
Upsetting another's Psychic vibrations."

She illustrated her poem by fanciful diagrams showing the interaction of various human radiations, their harmony or mutual interference. Her drawings looked so much like some of the illustrations that can be found in contemporary spiritualistic writings that it was difficult to establish her exclusive authorship of the pictures.

In the published work of such morbid geniuses as Swedenborg, the Seer of Stockholm, or August Strindberg, the writer, we are confronted with an analogous blend of method and madness, although on an incomparably higher plane. The origin of Swedenborg's teachings, culminating in his comprehensive mystical philosophy, has been ascribed to a paraphrenic process, as also has his account of his habitual intercourse with angels and spirits, of his glimpses of the " Unseen World ", and his claim to possess telepathic and clairvoyant powers. August Strindberg's psychosis shows unmistakable features of paranoic schizophrenia. In his autobiographic writings he gives a graphic description of his morbid hyper-sensitiveness to the demeanour of his fellow-men, to their facial expressions, to their secret thoughts and emotions. He depicts his vain attempt to " cloak himself in the silken coat of solitude " and to escape the painful presence of those around him. The final break-down of his married life was obviously precipitated by similar delusional experiences. He writes, with reference to his wife : " I could perceive the variations of her feelings from afar as an impression between taste and smell. . . . One night when she hated me I perceived the taste and smell of *mortaline* (a made-up word) so strong that it forced me to get up and open the window. On occasions when she thought lovingly of me I would perceive the perfume of incense or jessamine."

It is significant that he maintained his claim to possess some sort of occult powers also during his normal phases. " Child, the human thought needs no wires to make a way for itself from mind to mind. . . ." More recently, P. C. Squire devoted a special study to Strindberg's alleged psychic or clair-audient faculties.

But in whatever form the delusional ideas of the paranoic patient present themselves, whether in the guise of an elaborate philosophical system, of a fascinating work of art, or in the disjointed mutterings of a semi-demented patient, the interpretation offered by the modern psychological approach is certainly in flagrant contradiction to the patient's own reading. Indeed, the projection hypothesis of paranoic delusions, advanced by the psychoanalysts is nothing else than the reverse of the telepathy hypothesis, its photographic negative, as it were. It may be recalled that it was the autobiography of the paranoic Dr. Schreber that served as the point of departure of Freud's celebrated theory of paranoia. The place of telepathic influences in Dr. Schreber's case was taken by mysterious rays emanating from the Sun, a symbolic representation of Dr. Flechsig, the patient's physician. This honourable scientist he considered was the principal source of the unspeakable tortures which he had to endure. Freud's interpretation makes it clear that in actual fact the paranoic is tormented by his own sadistic-aggressive or homosexual tendencies originating from his unconscious. He is sensitive to what we called his auto-psychic material, not to influences emanating from his fellows. He projects his own repressed wishes and desires into the outer world.

This interpretation has been widely accepted by contemporary psychopathology and there can be little doubt that, besides giving a reasonable explanation of the patient's attitude, it is in good keeping with a wealth of observations derived from the field of clinical psychiatry and psychotherapy in general. On the o her hand, it must be admitted that the absurdity of the patient's interpretation seems to be immediately apparent. It is in fact the predominant feature of his mental disorder. This is also borne out by the natural reaction of the patient's friends and relations to his statements. In bygone times this reaction frequently assumed the form of merciless repressive measures or savage attempts at exorcising the evil spirits of which the patient was thought to be possessed. In our days this attitude is mitigated into scorn or ridicule which is meted out to him by the illiterate, or else to the indignation felt by common sense over his nonsense. However this may be, his friends and relations leave no doubt as to what they think of his phantastic allegations, and their views are readily endorsed by the certifying authorities. Indeed, is it not absurd to suggest that there should be a grain of truth in Strindberg's accusations of his unfortunate wife? Is it not ridiculous to state that Dr. Flechsig should in actual fact have harboured sadistic-aggressive tendencies against his paranoic patient? In short, is not any intimation of a telepathic reading of the case of paranoia likely to appear as a concession to the patient's own point of view and, therefore, itself suggestive of mental derangement?

There is a further argument which can be raised against a telepathic reading. We mentioned that psychoanalysis has revealed the reasons for man's clinging to certain concepts of magic and animism such as still survive in the obsessional practices of the compulsion neurotic, in the superstitions of the spiritualists and in some of the claims of psychical research. The psychoanalyst is indeed inclined to consider all these beliefs as further confirmations of Freud's thesis of the alleged "omnipotence of thought" as a characteristic feature of primitive mentality. Freud pointed out that there is still a tendency of the human mind to over-estimate psychic processes, as opposed to reality, and to force the laws which apply to man's inner experience upon the things of the outer world. Guided by this " intellectual narcism " he may believe that whatever he wishes to happen is going to happen as a matter of fact, and that " relations which exist between ideas exist also between things ". This is, on Freud's view, the mainspring of man's belief in telepathy. Telepathic phenomena are not, after all, facts that call for explanation. Belief in them is rather itself a symptom of regression to a primitive stage of mentality and as such in need of psychoanalytical inquiry. This was, at least, the view originally held by Freud before his conversion to a more receptive attitude towards the new facts revealed by psychical research.

Summing up, there are three chief objections to the application of the telepathy hypothesis to the problem of paranoia. First, the telepathy hypothesis closely resembles the patient's own reading of his case. This is by itself bound seriously to compromise the very sanity of its advocates. Secondly, the explanation offered by the projection hypothesis suggests precisely the opposite reading. Thirdly, it can be asserted that the telepathy hypothesis is itself nothing more than a product of morbid or primitive mentality.

But are these objections really conclusive? Cannot the fact that the telepathy hypothesis seems to tally with some of the patient's own illusions just as well indicate that his delusions are not completely irrational after all? Again, if the new reading is in flagrant contradiction to an old established theory, do not, one may argue, doubts referring to either theories cut both ways? Finally, if the psychoanalyst relegates all claims regarding the very existence of telepathic phenomena into the realm of phantasy and wishful thinking, he is given the lie by the mass of evidence which indisputably proves their occurrence. In short, arguments for or against the *prima facie* probability of the telepathy hypothesis as applied to our issue are inconclusive and amount to merely stating and re-stating two opposing points of view. Evidently the question can only be decided in the light of factual observations, afforded by comparative analysis of both the patient and his alleged persecutor.

* * * * * * *

In the first case to be reviewed here, the thankless role of an alleged persecutor fell to myself, whilst the patient, who may be called Leon A., was my playmate from early childhood. I can thus supplement his case history by the account of my own recollections of our mutual relationship. My first memory of Leon refers to an incident when he was four years old. I met him at a children's party when he fearfully hid himself in a corner. He was of a shy and timid disposition. In the following years he proved to be a mediocre student and a poor mixer, lacking self-reliance, drive and initiative. He had no intimate friends but showed, nevertheless, marked attachment to me and seemed eager to follow my example in various ways, which became increasingly apparent during his adolescent years. He had passed with difficulty his High School examinations and decided to go up to Prague to study medicine at the same medical school as myself. He took this step without informing me of his intention and I remember that I welcomed him with mixed feelings when he arrived there. I should mention here that part of the reason for my ambiguous reaction was that Leon was at that time financially dependent on my family and I did not consider his prospects in a medical career altogether favourable.

The first manifest symptoms of Leon's illness developed at that time. He disclosed to me that he was about to make a great discovery. He claimed that he had detected in himself the faculty of reading the thoughts of his fellow students and he complained that they were in turn able to influence him with their thoughts. In time these influences became more and more distressing and his mental condition increasingly alarming. I consulted Professor Alfred Pick in Prague on his behalf. He diagnosed a paranoid schizophrenia and recommended his admission to a mental hospital for which I made the necessary arrangements. Leon's attachment to his former friend soon yielded to bitter resentment. He wrote letter after letter imploring me to free him from his agonising experiences. The disturbing influences, he asserted, were now coming from me. He complained that I tormented him with an electric apparatus. The tone of his letters became increasingly menacing and hostile. It was clear that I had become his main persecutor, the central figure of his delusional system.

At first sight this course of Leon's illness seems to be in good keeping with the projection theory. Indeed, the whole setting of the case seems to bear some superficial resemblance to the psychological constellation in the case of Dr. Schreber and his physician. But while we can learn nothing from Freud's monograph about Dr. Flechsig's attitude towards his patient, it is possible in the present connection to make my own attitude towards Leon the object of closer inquiry.

I mentioned that in the course of his illness, Leon's attachment to the friend of his adolescent years had turned to hatred. I also intimated that as far as my own feelings were concerned they were not entirely free from a tinge of resentment though tempered by my sympathy for him in his misfortune. This ambivalent attitude was also illustrated by dreams which I regularly recorded at that time and in which he was repeatedly involved. The dreams cannot for obvious reasons be reproduced here in detail. Be it sufficient to remark that on several occasions they showed evidence of vague hostility towards him, following a trivial incident connected with a girl with whom we were both friendly.

So much about the psychological constellation in the case of Leon *versus* the present writer. What, then, is the relevance of this observation to our issue? Is it permissible to suggest on the ground of the available evidence that the patient's accusations were not entirely irrational after all? Did his paranoic trend contain a grain of truth, based on something like a selective sensitiveness of his deranged mind to unconscious aggressive tendencies of my own? And if so, is it permissible to assume that it is these vague and ill-defined complexes in my own mind which were reflected in his delusional ideas?

Obviously, such a far-reaching conclusion must remain a matter of conjecture. There undoubtedly is some correspondence between a certain trend of my unformulated thoughts concerning Leon, and between Leon's delusions relating to me. But this correspondence cannot be substantiated by reference to such well-defined data as may be encountered in successful experiments with freely chosen material, to say nothing of the usual card-calling tests.

The common denominator in the two series of mental events considered here is of an utterly non-specific nature. Unconscious, aggressive or sadistic-homosexual tendencies can easily be detected even in normal persons through deep psychological investigation. Indeed, psychoanalysts maintain that they are a regular feature of the human mind. But if this be true, it must also be admitted that the projection hypothesis which attributes the patient's ideas of persecution to his own repressed tendencies is likewise applicable to whomsoever is subjected to the same scrutiny. The correspondence between the paranoic's delusions and what here, too, may be described as his auto-psychic material, is by no means more compelling than the correspondence with what we termed hetero-psychic material. This means in other words that a substantial part of the evidence upon which the projection hypothesis is founded is in no way more conclusive than the evidence from which a telepathic reading can be derived. It is at bottom equally amenable to both interpretations.

A second group of observations refers to a married couple, Mr. and Mrs. P., with whom I had been on friendly terms for several years. Mr. P. was an architect, aged forty-two. His wife was an attractive woman aged thirty. One day Mr. P. consulted me about her and disclosed the tragedy of his married life. His wife suspected him of misconduct with his woman secretary and with some of her friends. She even maintained that he had sexual intercourse with his sister and claimed that she found visible proof of this in her bedroom. She described her life with her husband as a hell, complained of being neglected sexually, and insisted on immediate divorce. She was admitted to a mental hospital and had a temporary remission following insulin treatment.

Mr. P. responded to his wife's illness with a nervous breakdown. He developed a typical psychogenic depression with suicidal ideas. He underwent a short course of psychotherapy with me in which he declared that although Mrs. P.'s accusations were utterly without foundation he was guilty "in thought". "There was nothing between myself and my secretary, but I am afraid I noticed her presence in a way I should not have had to. You see, working so close together, day by day. . . ." The analysis of his dreams revealed a marked fixation on his sister, actually on the same one to whom his wife's morbid jealousy referred. Mr. P. soon realised the futility of his self-accusations and regained his mental balance.

In this case too, there is a striking correspondence between the principal motifs of the patient's paranoic trend on the one hand and a group of unconscious complexes in the mind of the person against whom her morbid suspicion is directed, on the other. The correspondence seems to be even more pronounced than in the previous case. Especially Mrs. P.'s delusions referring to her husband's incestuous relations dovetail in a striking manner with Mr. P.'s self-reproaches conditioned by his unconscious incestuous phantasies. However, even these far-reaching congruencies are open to objections. It can be argued that there may still have been some slight justification in Mrs. P.'s accusations, or that at least part of her husband's feeling of guilt, as well as the patient's delusions, were derived from essentially identical sources of the unconscious in which we are always likely to light upon identical symbols.

The following case confronts us with a further difficulty. One of my patients—a teacher in an elementary school—aged thirty, was rejected by the Education Committee when first applying for his post. He was told by his father that, in the view of Mr. N., the Chairman of the Committee, they regarded him as " daft ". The patient had in fact a marked paranoic disposition and following this incident he developed ideas of reference, focussed on the person of Mr. N. The patient considered this man his evil spirit, the destroyer of his life. Now, Mr. N., in contrast to the foregoing case, was not available for personal interrogation for the simple reason that he died shortly after the episode described. However, his death did by no means relieve the patient's persecutional trend. His hatred of the destroyer of his life remained unabated and his mental condition got gradually worse. In the further course he developed what psychoanalysts call a negative transference against me with a strong paranoic colouring and he broke up the treatment.

Clearly, this case cannot easily be reconciled with our tentative formulation of the telepathy hypothesis as applied to the paranoic reaction type. If it is true to say that the patient's paranoic attitude was due to what we called hetero-psychic sensitiveness, this sensitiveness must have extended beyond the range of the alleged unconscious aggressive tendencies in the mind of Mr. N. alone. It must be thought to cover a much wider range, embracing similar tendencies on the part of his father, of myself and of those in authority in general—indeed, of whomsoever he happened to identify with Mr. N. who was in turn no one else than a typical father representative in the psychoanalytical sense.

But it must be admitted here that even so our theory would rest on slender grounds so far as proofs are concerned. Here too, as in the case of the dream, or of the mediumistic trance, it is difficult to disentangle the respective part played by auto-psychic and hetero-psychic elements, and harder still to find out the relative importance of the two factors in the origin of the patient's negativistic reaction towards them. In our analysis of the cases reviewed here, we laid special stress on the patient's assumed sensitiveness to unconscious sadistic-aggressive tendencies of his friends and relations. But it is readily understood that unconscious tendencies of this kind, originating from a variety of agents, are of such a general, nondescript nature as to make their identification in the mind of an assumed percipient practically impossible. They lack all the criteria on which the claim of an unequivocal telepathic correspondence could be founded. To put it in other words : what correspondence our tentative comparative analysis of the patient and his alleged persecutor has revealed may or may not be of a telepathic nature, but the available evidence is equivocal and amenable both to the telepathic and to the more orthodox Freudian interpretation.

It will be noted, however, that this difficulty does not necessarily reflect upon the validity of our thesis. It is, in fact, largely due to the very nature of the material here discussed. In the chapter that follows we therefore propose to attack the problem from another angle and to review a series of observations made on patients of a different class from the point of view of the telepathy hypothesis.

Chapter IX

TELEPATHY AND SCHIZOPHRENIC DETERIORATION

THE observations discussed in the previous chapter were largely made in patients at the initial stages of the schizophrenic process, while they were still living in the community and able to follow their occupations in their ordinary environments. In the following pages we will review a series of observations in patients at a more advanced stage of the process, some having been confined in a mental hospital for a number of years. This means that both the clinical type of the patients and the whole psychological setting in which they were seen is totally different. The environment of an old inmate in a mental hospital is reduced to the standard conditions of institutional life. He gradually loses touch with the problems that confronted him in the outer world ; his friends and relations recede into the background and are replaced by his daily intercourse with fellow patients or with the medical and nursing staff.

Such a psychological setting has both advantages and disadvantages from the angle of our inquiry. Its advantages lie in the fact that the observer happens to play at the same time the part of the patient's principal social environment with the result that his comparative analysis can be based on observation of the patient on the one hand, and self-observation on the other. Its disadvantage lies in the fact that it imposes upon the observer a dual task. He has to focus his attention on his inner experience and combine this introspective attitude with the indispensable keen observation of the patient. This undoubtedly is a widely different approach from his routine hospital duties and requires experience in subtle psychological observation and self-observation which can only be acquired through years of training in psychotherapeutical work.

Even so, the difficulties of a systematic investigation are obvious. I pointed out that the conditions for the origin of telepathy are beyond the control of the experimenter. They are likely to occur precisely at moments when he is off his guard and unprepared to pay them the necessary attention. On the other hand, the phenomena will generally fail to materialise once his attention is focussed on them. This peculiar elusive behaviour of telepathic occurrences is particularly marked in schizophrenic patients under clinical conditions and anyone expecting to find them on his daily hospital round as a matter of routine may be sorely disappointed. In fact, my best observations in the present series occurred at a time when I was not at all in a suitable mood for scientific observation.

Unfortunately, reasons of privacy limit the extent to which personal references can be included in the material reviewed. I intimated that it is largely based on analysis of the patients' productions as compared with my own train of thought, conscious and pre-conscious, at the time of observation: but while I am at liberty to omit or include in this report a particular item at my own discretion, I have to exercise stricter censorship where the privacy of other persons is concerned. For this reason the institutions in which some of the observations were made cannot be divulged, and names, dates, and other particulars have to be altered. However, I may emphasise that the account of the actual observations is substantially accurate. It is based on verbatim notes taken after each occurrence. Further, in the majority of institutional cases I was able to have my records checked against the evidence of the ward sister, or another member of the staff who was present during the interviews.

The first patient in this series is Florence C., a schizophrenic at an advanced stage of the process with marked catatonic features. She is negativistic, given to impulsive outbursts, exposes herself and exhibits various mannerisms and antics. I first saw her on the 21st June 1942, shortly after I had commenced work in an institution new to me. I was about to make the routine six-monthly notes in her case-sheet and cast a brief glance at her particulars before proceeding to her side room. The case-sheet contained the usual data, such as her name, age, address, date of admission, etc. Admitted in 1935, she was thirty years of age at that time, that is to say, thirty-seven at the time of the interview. However, I mistook the significance of " 1935 " in a moment of absent-mindedness and jumped to the wrong conclusion that she was thirty-five years old, that is, seven years my junior. This mistake is perhaps better understood if I mention that having been born in 1900 I had made it a habit to calculate other persons' ages by comparing their birth-data with my own year of birth. After my casual glance at her papers I entered the patient's room and put the usual question : " How old are you ? " No answer. Wanders about the room, grimaces. " How old are you ? " " Don't ask silly questions . . . you are seven years older than me. . . ." No further conversation was possible. She took no notice of my presence and remained resistive to examination. Her apparent reference to the erroneous result of my calculation struck me only when I had left the patient. I returned to the ward and asked the Ward Sister whether she could remember the patient's remark. She confirmed the utterance recorded. Two months later I tried to draw the patient into another conversation. " How old are you ? " " Don't know ". " Are you married ? " " No, Spinster . . . You know ". Fidgets about. " Ask your own wife . . . and brother." Rambles incoherently. When questioned on other occasions she remained inaccessible and refused to answer.

The first reaction of this patient is undoubtedly significant. It contains a reference to a definite item, the presence of which at that time in my own mind I was able to establish with a reasonable degree of certainty. Further, her remark cannot reasonably be ascribed to a correct guess at my own age which she in reality misjudged. The fact is, that it exactly corresponds with the result of my own miscalculation in a moment of absent-mindedness. This point should be particularly noted. A correct estimate by the patient of my age would clearly be of lesser value, for it could then easily be explained as a lucky guess on her part, based on unconscious appreciation of sensory clues, rational inference, or the like. On the other hand, ascribing her reference to precisely seven years difference of age to chance alone is hardly justifiable, even though its improbability cannot be expressed in mathematical terms.

I may add a brief remark on her second reaction. The patient had referred to my wife and brother whom she advised me to question in her stead. Now it is true to say that I am married and have a brother who was actually living in my household at the time of the interview. But against this we have to note that the reference to a wife and a brother might well fit the description of every third or fourth person of my age. It can, therefore, just as well be attributed to a simple guess and is of little evidential value.

A second observation refers to Dicky S., aged twelve, a case of juvenile schizophrenia with marked intellectual impairment. He was admitted to the hospital as a mental defective but showed a variety of catatonic symptoms such as grimacing, tricks and mannerisms, as well as phases of emotional poverty, alternating with psychomotor restlessness and agitation. In the weeks following his admission I had almost lost sight of Dicky, and when I saw him again after two months I was struck by his changed facial expression. His features appeared to have become coarser and he seemed to have grown older in the intervening time. I was about to remark on this to the ward attendant when Dicky butted in, " Dicky has become grown-up . . . ". On questioning he was unable to give any explanation of his utterance. He refused to answer and retired into his shell. The attendant assured me that he never heard Dicky making a similar remark before.

In this observation the correspondence between the patient's production and my own train of thought is quite unmistakable. It is open only to the one objection, that it may possibly be due to misrepresentation on my own part of what happened " on my end " of the occurrence. However, it must be noted that the same objection can be raised to every account of facts observed. All scientific experience, medical, psychological or otherwise, is ultimately derived from sensory impressions that pass through a terminal stage of " introspection ". Unless we are prepared to accept the validity of such data, no method of research can hold its ground.

The same consideration applies to the following case. Deborah B., aged thirty-three, has been suffering from schizophrenia for ten years and her condition is gradually deteriorating. She is demented, negativistic and unable to converse rationally. Her habits are faulty and degraded. She had been in a semi-stuporous state for nearly two months when she first attracted my attention in the day room. Her face seemed to be new to me. I noticed her dark, expressive eyes, her long eyelashes. Also, I distinctly remember pondering whether the dark rings under her eyes were due to make-up—an idea which I at once dismissed. A further impression I have recorded is that I realised in a flash her Jewish appearance. I turned to the Ward Sister with some measure of surprise and asked: " Who is this girl? "

She told me her name. The patient grimaced, rambled in her usual manner: " Peroxide . . . Eyebrows . . . I am Miss Lipstick . . . There are many Gentiles here . . . Open bottle chloroform . . . You will win a prize for it . . . Piano . . . etc."

In this case the correspondence, if any, of the patient's utterances and of my own thoughts is much more involved than in the previous instance. There are several items which have to be considered, viz. her reference to *peroxide*, *eyebrows*, *Miss Lipstick*, to the *many Gentiles here*, and lastly to the *open bottle* of *chloroform* for which I am going to *win a prize*. Perhaps the eyebrow motif originated in the impression I had received from her eyes and eyelashes. On reflection, however, I cannot recall having particularly noticed her eyebrows. Her reference to peroxide can hardly be registered in the same group of associations and cannot, therefore, be accounted for. The same is true for the word " piano " which she uttered twice, unless we relate it to her previous interest in playing the piano. Her claim that she is Miss Lipstick, however, seems to lead back to my vague idea of make-up evoked by her appearance.

I now come to her reference to the many Gentiles here. This may be interpreted as a contrast-association to my impression of her Jewish features. Again, the motif of the prize-winning bottle can only be accounted for by free associations of my own. As a matter of fact, I did keep a bottle in my drawer, although it did not contain chloroform but a solution of ether and another substance which I used for experimental purposes. I was at that time greatly interested in the matter and believed that I had found a useful therapeutic mixture. This may possibly account for the motif of winning a prize for it. To this I may add that the bottle with ether—the sister substance of chloroform—was the only bottle I had among my belongings in my office and that on the day before when using the ether solution for disinfection, I nearly knocked it over, spilling part of its contents. I was a little concerned about the accident, and hesitated to ask the dispenser to make up the loss because I was reluctant to disclose the formula of my solution. This may possibly account for the patient's reference to an open bottle. So much about the bottle motif and its apparent relation to my free associations.

It will be noted that in this case the assumed correspondence between two " co-existent " series of mental events on the part of myself and the patient is of an indirect, symbolic or metaphorical nature, much less obvious than in the two previous observations. Indeed, none of Deborah's reactions can be regarded as a faithful reproduction of my own thoughts. They are near misses, scattered around a central idea of my own, in short, typical examples of what on an earlier page I described as telepathic scatter.

I was impressed by the patient's long eyelashes and noticed the bluish rings under her eyes. She produced the word " eyebrow ", which is in close topographic correlation with it. Likewise, her reference to " Miss Lipstick " is a close approximation to my general impression of make-up, of which lipstick assuredly is an integral part. Peroxide seems to be more remote from this idea though it might be argued that it, too, is loosely connected with the notion of make-up. The allusion to chloroform, which, according to my interpretation, actually stands for ether, is another near miss, whilst I already mentioned that the patient's reference to the many Gentiles here may be due to her being side-tracked into a chain of contrast-associations.

It will be recalled that in the view of E. Bleuler this kind of side-tracking of associations is a fundamental feature of schizophrenic thinking. Alfred Storch has further elaborated this thesis. He stressed the close similarity of schizophrenic thought to thought in primitive races and children. Their ideas are not made up of well-defined concepts. They consist of vague, symbol-like or complex representations in which one component part may stand for the whole, and *vice versa*. More recent investigators described the impairment of conceptual thinking in schizophrenics along similar lines.

If this is true, it will be readily understood that the schizophrenic disorder of thinking may itself be conducive to much the same tendency to scatter of associations as is characteristic of telepathy. It is interesting to note that in this respect the colloquial description of certain schizophrenic border-line cases and eccentrics as *scatterbrains* seems to hit the nail on the head.

In the following observation a young medical student played the part of the agent, whilst the part of the percipient was played by George H., aged sixty, a patient suffering from a paraphrenic psychosis, complicated by occasional epileptic fits. George H.'s delusions were of an expansive religious kind. He claimed that he was under the direct command of the Lord, that he was in charge of the hospital and that God had bestowed on him the gift of divination. He was a man of the working class with very limited educational attainments, but he used to tell the "fortunes" of his interviewers in a bizarre and grandiose fashion, applying more or less ready-made clichées in the manner of Market Place palmists or astrologers, yet sometimes striking surprisingly individual notes. "You are not a doctor", he said one day to the young student. "You are Mr. Daniel. You have been living with a woman to whom you are not married. She has two children and you deserted her and her children when you took this job. . . ."

On this I have to remark that the young man had in actual fact entertained a friendship with an attractive divorced woman, a mother of two children. It need not be emphasised that only a few of his friends were aware of this attachment. The young man recounted to me the patient's remark as a mere curiosity, without realising its apparent relevance to his own case. He was deeply struck when I offered him my interpretation. Two weeks after the incident described, he gave notice and left his place of employment as well as his friend and her two children. He confessed to me that at the time of the interview with the patient he was already contemplating leaving the hospital and breaking up his attachment.

I mentioned that the patient had a variety of stereotyped patterns after which his utterances were fashioned. This may be illustrated by a brief account of an interview which I had with him soon after the above-mentioned episode.

"You are not a doctor", he said, "you only pretend to

be a doctor. Your father is a Japanese, your mother is a Belgian . . . Your salary is eight pounds but you have to give three pounds to the relieving officer."

It need not be observed that these confabulations have no bearing upon facts.

However, in the case of the alleged Mr. Daniel, the correspondence between certain facts of the young man's "secret life" and the patient's statement is quite unmistakable. There is, firstly, the reference to his attachment to a married woman; secondly, to the fact that she was mother of two children; thirdly, to his having abandoned her. These three references show such a striking correlation with the actual facts that they cannot reasonably be ascribed to chance alone. However, the third point requires comment. It will be noted that the patient referred to Mr. Daniel's faithlessness as to an episode in his past life history, whereas he in reality anticipated his intended step. But this apparent inconsistency by no means impairs the significance of his reaction. We know from the analysis of dreams that past, present and future have no real meaning to the unconscious. It was obviously only a matter of chance that he failed to couch his statement in terms of a prediction of future events. Had he done so, it would have appeared more striking still and even more reminiscent of the attempted prophecies of professional fortune-tellers and astrologers.

I may recall at this point the telepathic interpretation of the Weird Sisters prophecy, predicting Macbeth's rise to power to which I referred in Chapter IV. I suggested that the witches were in actual fact sensitive to Macbeth's secret desire to become Thane of Cawdor, Thane of Glamis and King Duncan's successor, whatever the price, although he himself was largely unaware of the sinister designs that were looming at the back of his mind. Precisely the same interpretation suggests itself to George H.'s utterance. He, too, did little more than reflect in a telepathic way the young man's secret thoughts, as yet unformulated, and in *statu nascendi*, so to speak, but carrying in themselves the germ of his future actions.

The patient's reaction confronts us in this way once more with the problem of the time factor in telepathy. I emphasised in Chapter IV the difficulty of determining the temporal coincidence of two series of mental events in terms of physical simultaneousness. I pointed out that on closer examination some measure of temporal discrepancy, of a time lag, positive or negative, is invariably present in phenomena of this kind, adding that this state of affairs can well be accounted for by the scatter theory which substitutes for chronological simultaneity the psychological recency or topicality of the mental events concerned.

The theory of telepathic scatter thus helps us to overcome one of the most intriguing implications of telepathy, experimental and spontaneous. It gives us the common denominator of both types of phenomena, whether observed in the laboratory, under clinical conditions, or whether they were conceived by the imagination of the creative artist. At the same time, it relieves us from the task of deciding the difficult question whether or not true pre-cognitive telepathy has taken place in a concrete case, or it makes such a decision at least irrelevant to our issue.

However, the existence of telepathic scatter, thus conceived, confronts us with a new difficulty which has so far escaped our attention. It makes the notion of telepathy unduly elastic, so to speak ; it is apt to overstrain its meaning. Indeed, unless we arrive at an understanding regarding the period of time which we are prepared to allow for its operation, there would be no limit set to the range of telepathic scatter, and we should be faced with the impossible task of comparing two, theoretically speaking, infinite series of mental events (stretching into a boundless past and future) regarding the incidence of telepathic occurrences. The discussion of the intriguing philosophical implications of such a proposition would go far beyond the scope of our inquiry. I may only remark that they have puzzled some of the critics of Dunne's *Experiment with Time* whose pre-cognitive interpretation of dreams involves much the same problem and they have added to the difficulties of the statistical appreciation of such pre-cognitive and post-cognitive reactions as were found in Whately Carington's drawing tests or in the Soal-Goldney card-calling experiments.

As far as the appreciation of spontaneous observations is concerned, there is only one way to evade the difficulties attached to the theoretically unlimited range of telepathic scatter. We must agree on a conventional time limit beyond which we refrain from extending considerations. My own experience has shown that this period should be not more than twenty-four hours and that the evidence in cases implying a greater temporal discrepancy is usually open to so many objections as to make it inconclusive.

There is a further difficulty which seems to be inherent in our method. We pointed out that our evidence is largely derived from comparative analysis of the patient's utterances on the one hand, and of the observer's introspections on the other. But it should not be overlooked that this, too, is an entirely arbitrary restriction of our frame of reference. We have no reason to preclude the possibility of other quasi-telepathic influences affecting the patient's mind in a similar way. Patient and observer are not operating in a psychological vacuum. I mentioned that most of the observations to which I referred were made with the Ward Sister or other members of the staff present; in some cases in wards with occupants averaging between forty and fifty patients, to say nothing of their friends and relations, their visitors and other contacts, past and prospective. However, it is clear that we have no means to find out whether, and how far, latent influences from these sources are involved in the patient's productions. What we called comparative analysis of the total situation is thus—strictly speaking—beyond our reach, and we must be satisfied with its nearest approximation.

It is, perhaps, these perplexities of both theory and practice, coupled with our ingrained fear of the irrational, which explain why the telepathic factor involved in the productions of schizophrenic patients has so long escaped our notice. On the other hand, it must be admitted that even the full exploitation of the available evidence in the field of abnormal psychology has yielded only a limited harvest of indisputably telepathic observations in schizophrenics. However, it has become an acknowledged principle of psychical research at its present stage that it is not the number but the quality of the observations which decides the issue. Such reactions as those recorded in Florence C., or Dicky S., are as conclusive as spontaneous phenomena can be, and some of Deborah B.'s utterances are not less significant. They suggest that the occurrence of telepathy in patients of this group can no longer be denied.

What then, is the significance of these findings? I have to recall here what I said in Chapter VI about the part played by telepathy in the psychoanalytic situation. I pointed out that whenever we are satisfied with the possibility of telepathic influences becoming operative from the analyst to the patient or from the patient to the analyst in a small way, it is only fair to assume that their cumulative effect may make itself felt also in a large way. Precisely the same applies to the case of our schizophrenics. If the patient shows evidence of hetero-psychic sensitiveness to such trivial items as my miscalculation of her age, or to my vague impression of " make-up ", we can hardly escape the conclusion that the same sort of sensitiveness may be responsible for reactions which have more direct bearing upon the under-lying process. In short, we must assume that on the strength of the same hypothesis, hetero-psychic material of a more relevant type may become telepathically active on the patient's mind. This precisely is the tentative result of the argument pursued in the previous chapter.

Indeed, when discussing the part played by the telepathic factor at earlier stages of the schizophrenic process we pointed out that there is a great deal of circumstantial evidence available to suggest such a possibility, although we had to add that none of the cases reviewed in the paranoic group yielded unequivocal clues in this respect. Seen against the background of the paranoic reaction type the importance of the trivial observations reviewed in the present chapter is obvious. They suggest that what happened in patients at an advanced stage of the process might also occur in patients at an earlier stage.

But is such an argument by analogy really justified? Is it fair to assume that the patients reviewed in the two foregoing chapters are of the same clinical type? And is it permissible to suggest that the two instances of hetero-psychic sensitiveness, referring as they do to two different patterns of hetero-psychic material, can be considered under a common heading? In short, has the evidence reviewed in this section any bearing upon the hypothesis put forward in the previous chapter? We will try to answer this question in the chapter that follows by joining together the two separate strands of our argument.

10

Chapter X

THE TELEPATHY HYPOTHESIS AND THE CLINICAL PICTURE OF SCHIZOPHRENIA

THE questions put at the end of the previous chapter call for a statement of facts well-known to the medical reader. He may, therefore, just as well skip the next paragraph or two. However, for the sake of the non-medical reader I may remark that the correlation between paranoia and what we described as schizophrenic deterioration is not merely accidental. We know that as a general rule a great proportion of patients exhibiting ideas of persecution or reference—that is, paranoic features—tend to develop into true schizophrenics with all the symptoms of gradual disintegration of their personalities. On the other hand, it is an established fact that most schizophrenics at an advanced stage of the process have passed through a paranoic phase at an earlier stage of their illness.

This, for instance, is the case in most of the patients to whom I referred on previous pages. Leon A., the medical student whose paranoic psychosis I described, developed into a typical demented schizophrenic in the ensuing years. On the other hand, the early histories of Florence C., and Deborah B., reveal that their illnesses were ushered in by a typical paranoic trend with ideas of reference and persecution. In fact, this correlation between two consecutive stages of the schizophrenic process, has been the chief argument in favour of Kraepelin's older conception of dementia paranoides, or more recently, Bleuler's paranoic schizophrenia. We can therefore rely on good authority in classing the patients discussed in the previous sections in one common clinical group.

But are we equally justified in assuming that there exists a similar correlation between the two types of hetero-psychic sensitiveness in the patients reviewed in the two foregoing chapters? It will be recalled that in discussing the telepathic interpretation of the paranoic reaction type, our argument was based on the assumption that the paranoic may be sensitive to unconscious or repressed sadistic-aggressive tendencies of his fellows, whilst patients at an advanced stage of the process showed no indication of hetero-psychic sensitiveness to influences of this kind. On the other hand, we failed to detect signs of telepathic sensitiveness in paranoic patients to hetero-psychic influences emerging from the pre-conscious sphere. To this we may add in passing only that, in a similar vein, card-calling tests carried out in the U.S.A. on patients of the paranoic group showed no evidence of extra-chance scoring.

This would seem to indicate that such telepathic sensitiveness as exists in the two groups refers to two separate things, or at least that the patients may be susceptible to two entirely different patterns of hetero-psychic influences at the two successive stages of the process. However, the following observation shows that such an artificial discrimination is hardly justifiable.

Catherine J., aged twenty-four, a schizophrenic with marked paranoic features watched a fellow-patient of about her own age, Betty H., breaking out of her side-room, smashing a window pane and sustaining slight cuts to her wrist which necessitated stitching. Betty was a difficult patient and had failed to respond to insulin shock treatment. The day before I had remarked to the Ward Sister that I felt even my cautious attempts at humouring her might have had a paradoxical effect and only helped to bring about her recent relapse. After having attended to her wounds I found Catherine J., waiting for me in front of the side-room door. Reproachfully she turned to me: "*You* have done that to her. . . . *You* made her do it!"

She ignored my explanations and maintained her charge. "You should have the courage to admit that you have made her do it. Why don't you admit it?"

The telepathic interpretation of this case is open to the usual objections. But accepting it for the sake of argument we would have to assume that in Catherine's case it was an ill-founded (though psychologically intelligible) feeling of guilt on my part which was "sensed" and promptly reproduced by the patient. If this is true it can be argued that the patient was sensitive, (1) to deeply repressed sadistic-aggressive material, (2) to mental contents of a less primitive kind, based on my pre-conscious feeling of guilt towards her. In this respect, her case is closely related to the case of Mrs. P., described in Chapter VIII, whose paranoic jealousy seemed to dovetail into her husband's feeling of guilt over his unconscious fixation on his sister.

Observations like these fill a gap in the evidence reviewed so far. They suggest that there may exist all grades and shades, indeed an infinite variety, of hetero-psychic sensitiveness, ranging from sensitiveness to very primitive, deeply repressed material of sadistic-aggressive kind to more highly differentiated influences, originating from pre-conscious strata of the agent's mind. It is interesting to note in this connection that from the psychiatric point of view, Catherine J. was a patient at a transitional stage of the schizophrenic process. In the further course, her paranoic trend became increasingly incoherent and she gradually passed into the terminal phase of schizophrenia.

It may be objected at this point that there is no evidence that the deterioration of her condition was in actual fact coupled with an extension of her range of hetero-psychic sensitiveness. But the absence of observations to this effect cannot be used as a proof in either direction. More important still, we already pointed out that most patients to whom we referred so far displayed a definite paranoic trend at the initial stages of their illnesses and that, conversely, closer observation of patients at a more advanced stage of the process invariably shows traces of a persisting paranoic trend. Even such deteriorated schizophrenics as Florence C., or Deborah B., leave us in no doubt that their fundamental attitude towards life has remained the same as at the height of their paranoic phase. They refuse to answer when spoken to; they are anxious to avoid any and every contact with their fellows; they are resistive to attention and may add injury to insult to anyone who would insist on trespassing on their privacy. This is what the textbooks of psychiatry describe as catatonic negativism in schizophrenic patients.

Viewed from our angle this catatonic negativism is by no means a senseless or irrational reaction. It is nothing else than the direct continuation on a reduced level of mentality of the patient's original attitude towards his delusional experiences, a direct derivative of, if not an equivalent to, the preceding paranoic phase. Put in terms of the telepathy hypothesis, this means that even at the stage of schizophrenic deterioration he has not in effect ceased to be sensitive to hetero-psychic influences of the sadistic-aggressive type and that his apparently irrational behaviour is in fact largely due to his desperate attempts to ward off and fight against his uncanny experiences, to shield himself against all conceivable human interference with his life, indeed against any and every relationship with his environment which he cannot help feeling menacing and wrought with danger.

An alternative reaction is the so-called catatonic stupor. The patient may be overwhelmed by the impact of a chaotic welter of hetero-psychic influences ; he may be paralysed by fear, like the rabbit in Kirchner's *experimentum mirabile*, he may respond with, physiologically speaking, a refractory phase to excessive stimulation. However, here again, all his efforts are unavailing. We can sometimes learn from patients recovering from catatonic stupor that their attempted escape from the maddening influx of stimuli from both the auto-psychic and the hetero-psychic sphere failed to bring relief. On the contrary, the patient, with his higher intellectual functions in abeyance, is more than ever exposed to the uprush of unconscious material from deeper strata, a vicious circle may be set up until his forces of resistance are spent and the terminal phase of his illness leads to the final break-down of his personality.

Another peculiar feature of catatonic schizophrenia is what psychiatrists describe as command-automatism, that is, stereotype movements or postures which the patient himself attributes to forces in the outer world, to a will alien to his own, acting upon his bodily functions. It is impossible to decide on the ground of the available evidence whether there is a grain of truth in this interpretation. But it is readily understood that an indirect effect of hetero-psychic influence upon the motor behaviour of a percipient would be in good keeping with the telepathy hypothesis. Indeed, it is a striking fact that there seems to be far-reaching agreement between the familiar accounts of various motor automatisms observed in trance mediums and the symptoms in catatonic patients.

There is a further aspect of the clinical picture of schizophrenia which calls for comment: the familiar case of the paranoic with ideas of grandeur. Patients of this type are strangely elated; they feel their vitality increased; their personality enriched; their inner senses expanded in an unheard-of manner. They boast of super-human powers of thought and perception and it is these cases which are most persistent in their claims of possessing telepathic, clairvoyant or mediumistic faculties. This picture has been largely attributed to the patient's narcissistic trend to self-elevation, associated with the withdrawal of libido from the outer world and by the influx of emotionally charged archaic material from the auto-psychic sphere. This interpretation is undoubtedly well justified, but it considers only one side of the picture and here, again, it can well be argued that auto-psychic sources are supplemented and enriched by hetero-psychic material which, in patients of this group, fails to assume the ominous negative feeling tone characteristic of most cases of paranoia.

In other patients again, the impact of indescribable, superhuman experiences may be registered in a mood of religious ecstasy, with a feeling of mystic union with the universe, with Heaven and Hell, as one of my patients put it, unwittingly quoting the title and prevailing theme of one of Swedenborg's writings. The productions of such patients may then show close correlation with mystic enlightenment, with the raptures and ecstasies of the saints; they may resemble the dramatic experience of the *mort mystique*, described by medieval ascetics; or else such spectacular states of trance as are brought about by the practices of the Yogis. This last point is all the more remarkable on recalling that A. Storch drew attention to the similarity of these states to conditions of catatonic stupor, and that the notorious Yoga-sleep has in turn been widely associated by popular belief both in the East and in the West with a variety of alleged supernormal phenomena.

In a last group of patients a very short paranoic phase may usher in the experience of a cosmic catastrophe, of the "end of the world". Terrifying hallucinations, emerging from chiefly auto-psychic sources, may culminate in a state of delirium or confusion, followed by a break-down and disintegration of the personality. At this stage the boundaries of the self are abolished, " the distinction between the ego and the environment suspended " (Jaspers) ; the patient may himself complain that he is unable "to tell himself from the outer world" (Storch), or from " things of the outer world " (Schilder). Seen from the angle of the telepathy hypothesis this state marks the end of the patient's struggle to maintain his personality against the impact of hetero-psychic influences of both sadistic-aggressive and trivial kind. If at an early stage of his illness his delusional trend was confined to selective sensitiveness to more or less specific patterns of auto-psychic or hetero-psychic material, the terminal phase is marked by the unchecked intrusion into what is left from his consciousness of a shapeless jumble of impressions from *both* spheres. It is the outcome of the complete break-down of the higher mental functions whose business it apparently is to safeguard the normal personality against this very predicament.

There can be little doubt that this tentative interpretation of the clinical picture of schizophrenia in the light of the telepathy hypothesis gives a reasonable account both of the familiar course and of the principal features of the process. But it leaves one question out of account : the question of causation. It does not explain why and in what way the patient develops his assumed telepathic sensitiveness to hetero-psychic material, first of sadistic-aggressive, and later of a more generalised, non-specific type. In this respect we have to rely on the interpretation given by the modern psycho-biological approach along more orthodox lines. I may only mention A. Meyer, F. Mott, and, more recently, R. E. Hemphill who called attention to the part played by neuro-glandular and metabolic disorders affecting the anatomical structure of the brain cortex, whilst Kretschmer's pioneer work opened our eyes to the striking correlation which exists between the patient's physical make-up and his characterological abnormalities.

We already briefly referred to the importance of the characterological factors from our point of view, and contrasted the negativistic attitude of the paranoic patient towards hetero-psychic experiences with the indulgent attitude of persons of the so-called psychic or hysteric type. But this is obviously only one side of the picture. There is a consensus of opinion on a characterological feature of a different order which is common to persons of the paranoic and schizophrenic reaction type. A. Hoch emphasises that paranoic schizophrenics have been abnormal personalities from the outset. He describes them as " persons who do not have a natural tendency to be open and get into contact with the environment, who are reticent, seclusive, who cannot adapt themselves to situations, who are hard to influence ", in short, are shut-in personalities.

The same characteristics are referred to by Bleuler's description of the schizophrenics as self-centred, autistic individuals ; by Freud's emphasis on their narcissistic libido organisation, or by Jung's formulation of the schizophrenic as the prototype of the introvert personality. Kretschmer, likewise, calls attention to the patient's difficulty in contact-finding, which he describes in terms of a peculiar anesthesia to human relationships which is in turn apt to enter into a paradoxical blend with the notorious hyper-sensitiveness of the schizophrenic. McDougall went so far as to consider the patient's faulty attitude towards his social environment, his lack of emotional contact and rapport as the principal feature of his abnormality. Indeed, there can be no doubt that this is a characteristic upon which all investigators are agreed.

On recalling our thesis of the presumable conditioning factors of telepathy in general, the relevance of this peculiar characterological disposition is obvious. Indeed, it seems to hold the key to the problem of causation in the psychological sphere. We pointed out that under otherwise favourable circumstances, telepathy may be due to a compensation of what we called a primary minus-function. We illustrated this point by Neureiter's case of Ilga K., the child suffering from congenital word-blindness, in whom an unusual telepathic reading ability was observed. Precisely the same mechanism may be involved in the case of the abnormal characterological make-up of the paranoid schizophrenic. If it is true that the patient is suffering from an intrinsic lack of rapport and emotional contact with his friends and relations, his delusional trend can rightly be described as an attempt to make up for his shortcomings by setting up a luxuriant system of imaginary relationships with his fellow-men. This delusional system fills a gap, as it were, in his notion of their attitudes towards him, and in so doing disposes of the last scruples he may entertain about them. He is now perfectly sure that they are against him, that he is surrounded by enemies, that he must be on his guard. It is obviously having regard to this tendency that A. Meyer described the schizophrenic process as a " miscarriage of the remedial work of life, just as fever, from being a self-defence, may become a danger and more destructive than its source ". But there is only one step from this formulation to the interpretation which is suggested by the telepathy hypothesis. Meyer attributes the schizophrenic process to a miscarriage of the remedial work of life, that is to say, to an over-compensation of the patient's primary defect along lines familiar in health and disease. Viewed from our angle, this tendency does not stop at that point. It is carried beyond the limitations of our established scientific experience into a sphere which has not so far been recognised by clinical psychiatry, though it will be noticed that it does not otherwise conflict with acknowledged biological principles.

However this may be, the evidence reviewed in the foregoing chapters shows that the telepathic factor plays an important part in the origin of the paranoic reaction type and, in the further course, in the development of such familiar symptoms as catatonic negativism, catatonic stupor, command-automatisms, etc. But it may be as well to note at this point that hetero-psychic influences represent only one part of, if not a fraction of, the primitive material which may impinge upon the patient's mind. In the view advanced by Bleuler, Jung and Storch, the schizophrenic process opens the door, as it were, to the impact of deeply repressed emotional complexes from what we have termed the auto-psychic sphere. They do not consider the feasibility of hetero-psychic influences, although it will be noted that Jung and, more recently, H. J. Baynes, stressed the role of the *collective unconscious* in the causation of the schizophrenic disorder. Jung pointed out that whenever the barriers which protect the integrity of the personality are impaired, primitive architypal elements, " the renegade forces of the soul " may break into the conscious sphere, disrupting the unity of the self and causing it to submerge in the rising tide of impersonal or supra-personal psychic experience.

In effect, our thesis amounts only to an amplification of this doctrine, suggested by the introduction of the telepathic factor into our argument. This is not meant to indicate that the clinical picture of schizophrenia is exclusively (or even predominantly) due to hetero-psychic influences. We hold that it is the result of the intrusion into the patient's consciousness of primitive material from *both* the auto-psychic and the hetero-psychic sphere, and to his individual reaction to this alarming experience. I may recall that in discussing the occurrence of telepathy in dreams we arrived at largely the same proposition. We found that the intricate fabric of the manifest dream content is likewise made up of auto-psychic material, interwoven with hetero-psychic elements. This fact gains added significance if we bear in mind the close correspondence which exists between the psychology of dreams and schizophrenia, the realisation of which has actually been one of the basic principles of the modern medico-psychological approach.

To sum up, the telepathic interpretation of the schizophrenic reaction type throws fresh light upon the clinical picture of the disease itself; it gives a fuller account of its familiar course than the orthodox school of thought, and it explains at the same time the various clinical manifestations of the disorder as diverse patterns of the patient's reaction to his auto-psychic and hetero-psychic experiences. In so doing, it links up the facts revealed with both the modern psychobiological approach and with our newly gained information about the part played by the telepathic factor in general.

But beyond this the telepathy hypothesis gives a reasonable account of the patient's apparently irrational behaviour, of the striking blend of method and madness presented by his paranoic trend, and it renders his " unshakable and irrectifiable delusional system " (Kraepelin) more intelligible. Indeed, it may be objected that undue emphasis on the telepathic reading might easily be misapprehended as an attempted exoneration of the patient's ideas, inconsistent as they are with ordinary common sense. But in order to dispel any possible misrepresentation, it may be emphasised that our thesis suggests nothing of this sort. If we stated that the paranoic is sensitive to repressed sadistic-aggressive tendencies of his fellow-men, we have to add that, for all practical intents and purposes, these tendencies remain none the less virtually non-existent. It is only through the patient's characterological defect that they are being invested with a semblance of life ; like Banquo's ghost they are visible to Macbeth's vexed imagination only.

On the other hand, the patient's reaction only confirms facts well known to psychoanalysis. We have learned from Freud that most of our emotions are made up of a compound of hatred and love, as water is made up of H_2 and O. We have learned to separate the two by means of psychological analysis, much in the same way as the analytical chemist contrives to break up the molecule of water into its component parts. It is the lot of the paranoic patient unwittingly to do the same sort of thing to the mental contents of his friends and relations. But in so doing, he cannot help losing his grip of the real world. Water is not just H_2 and O. Human relationships are not just a blend of hatred and love ; not only a struggle between Eros and Thanatos, between the instincts of procreation and destruction. This is why the patient's interpretation of life is doomed to failure ; and this is also why our new reading, unorthodox though it may be, arrives at much the same conclusions in point of biological evaluation as are commonly accepted by the man in the street.

However, it will be noted that at the same time it amounts to a remarkable vindication of the peculiar ambiguous attitude of the ancients towards what they described as demoniacal possession, as the sacred raptures of their prophets and saints, or as the unholy frenzies of their lunatics. Obviously, their attitude was determined by an intuitive realisation of both the veiled intimation of a transcendental psychic reality contained in these manifestations, and of their biologically incongruous character—of what Darwinists would call their negative survival value.

But it is clear that a truly rational approach has to refrain from bias in either direction. We may recall Hippocrate's famous verdict on epilepsy the " sacred disease ". " This disease ", he said, " is no more divine than any other disease. It has the same nature as any other diseases." It has been stated that this assertion marked the beginning of the modern era of psychiatry. However, our rational attitude should not lead to blinding ourselves to the existence of an irrational element in the borderland between sanity and mental illness, particularly in the group of mental disorders discussed here. On the contrary, it should be taken as a challenge to its proper appreciation within the context of our scientific world outlook, so as to fill the gaps which have so far remained in it. Telepathy and related phenomena may be at bottom atavistic functions of the human mind due to the re-emergence of obsolete patterns of psychic experience. Human society may rightly disapprove of their threatened reappearance on the level of waking consciousness. Indeed, it has gone so far as to repudiate every intimation of their very existence. But this should not relieve us of the responsibility to realise that they have not, nevertheless, ceased to occupy a place in our mental organisation, even though this place happens to be in precarious vicinity of mental derangement.

A brief remark may be appended on questions of treatment. The modern methods of shock and convulsion therapy are undoubtedly the most effective means of attacking the core of the disease, although their *modus operandi* has remained largely controversial. Here too, their appreciation in the light of the telepathy hypothesis may throw light on the problem. If we are right in assuming that the patient's delusional trend—and his hetero-psychic sensitiveness—are due to the over-compensation of a minus-function, brought about by the release of primitive strata of the central nervous system, it is reasonable to suggest that our therapeutic approach should proceed along two alternative lines. We may try to help the patient to make up for his primary defect, to restore his loosening grip on the world, to re-establish his emotional contact and rapport with his social environment. This can be achieved through psychotherapy along lines which are tacitly implied by our new interpretation. Or else we may try to attack the neuro-physiological mechanism which is responsible for the mobilisation of his faulty tendencies to compensation, to knock out, as it were, the anatomical structures upon which his abnormal hetero-psychic sensitiveness is hinged. This is apparently being done by the drastic methods of the modern psychiatric treatment. We know very little about the localisation and nature of the anatomical structures thus attacked, but it may well be that a deeper insight into the neuro-physiological and pathological aspects of the schizophrenic reaction type (and of the methods applied for its treatment) will give us at least a tentative clue in this direction.

PART IV

FRESH LIGHT ON CHARACTER AND PERSONALITY

Chapter XI

PORTRAIT OF A "PSYCHIC", CASE 1

We have seen in the foregoing chapters that in the long run the massive intrusion of hetero-psychic experiences into a person's mind may lead to the blunting of his mental functions and result in the final disintegration of his personality. We hinted that the principal characteristics of the paranoic reaction type can be expressed in terms of an increased sensitiveness to experiences of this kind and of the patient's frantic attempt to shield himself against their impact into his consciousness. To this we added that he may respond in much the same way to the " return of the repressed " from what we called the auto-psychic sphere and that this habitual reaction may be largely responsible for the fundamental attitude of the paranoic towards his social environment. Expressed in such terms this may appear as a somewhat unorthodox formulation, but it is in good keeping with the results of the modern characterological approach introduced by E. Kretschmer.

However, Kretschmer emphasised that the full-fledged picture of schizophrenia, leading to the gradual deterioration of the personality, represents an extreme case only. Persons of the so-called schizoid type may exhibit most of the characterological features of true schizophrenics yet always keep this side of the borderline of mental disorder. Again, Kretschmer's schizothymics are but a common variety of the normal characterological make-up, although in case of mental disorder they may be particularly prone to schizophrenic psychoses. Another group of persons belonging to the same characterological type may actually develop transient paranoic states with all the symptoms of paranoid schizophrenia, but usually regain their balance after a brief period of illness. A further group may exhibit the picture of expansive delusions of a religious kind with bizarre ideas of grandeur to which they cling with unshakable conviction and to which they may be able to convert a devoted band of disciples. But apart from their delusional trend they may preserve a remarkable degree of sanity and even exhibit features of genius, until their eccentric behaviour—or an impulsive act—may bring them into conflict with the authorities and lead to their confinement in an asylum. Kraepelin described this type as the group of paraphrenics and considered them as closely related with true paranoia and so-called dementia paranoides. However, Kretschmer rightly pointed out that, as a general rule, their characterological make-up is different and overlaps with features found in the manic-depressive or cyclothymic reaction type.

The paraphrenic group is of special interest in the present connection because academic psychiatry is inclined to class most eccentric personalities who claim to possess mediumistic faculties under this heading or at least as cases of so-called spiritualistic psychoses with paraphrenic features. A classical example of this is Emanuel Swedenborg, the Seer of Stockholm, one of the most original thinkers of his time, a universal genius whose interests ranged over the whole compass of seventeenth and eighteenth-century science and philosophy. Swedenborg was equally conversant with the teachings of Newton, Halley and Flamsteed as with the works of Spenser, Milton and Shakespeare. He was a pioneer in astronomy, geology and physics, and the originality of his studies in anatomy and physiology of the central nervous system, particularly of the cerebro-spinal fluid and the ductless glands have been acknowledged by such an authority in anatomy as Retzius. In a different branch of science he gave a lucid account of the phenomena of phosphorescence and propounded a nebular theory of the universe, closely resembling modern physical concepts. Indeed, Professor Herbert Dingle pointed out that some of the ideas of Einstein's physical world have been foreshadowed in Swedenborg's writings as early as 1734. Especially his celebrated *Principia* show, to quote Professor Dingle, " the tremendous intellectual power of a man who, without the guidance needed by many of the best minds of to-day could attain to conceptions essentially identical with those of our most advanced scientific theories ".

In addition to these activities he tried his hand at a variety of inventions. He described a *New Method of Finding the Longitude* and is said to have designed a flying machine and a submarine. He travelled widely on the Continent, edited a scientific journal, was assessor of the Swedish Board of Mines and a member of the Swedish House of Nobles. But the striking fact is that the same man, at the age of fifty-seven, under the influence of a " mystic illumination ", abandoned all his worldly interests and for the rest of his life devoted himself to writing his countless volumes of theological and metaphysical works. " I have been called to a holy office by the Lord ", he declared, " who most graciously manifested Himself before me, His servant, in the year 1745, and opened my sight into the spirit world and gave me to speak with spirits and angels as I even do to-day." In writing this he is well aware that " many persons will insist that this is impossible and that such an intercourse must be mere fancy, or that I have invented such relations in order to gain credit for my doctrines ". But he adds : " For all these I do not care, for I have seen, heard and felt ".

His claims were not confined to mystic revelations from the Lord only ; he also maintained that he was able to communicate with the souls of the deceased, with spirits dwelling on the moon and other planets. " If one spirit desires to see another, this desire instantly brings them together." In addition, he claimed to possess what would now be called clairvoyant powers, and his earlier biographers state that in one of his visions he actually gave a correct description of a fire that raged at Stockholm while he was many miles away. But they also remark that from the time of his conversion onward his mind grew " morbidly hypochondriacal " and his behaviour increasingly eccentric.

Swedenborg has gained wide reputation both as a pioneer of science and as a religious mystic. A considerable number of his followers and scores of Swedenborg Societies in various countries, headed by the so-called New Church, still adhere to his teachings, but from the angle of clinical psychiatry there can be little doubt that he must be classed as a morbid genius, presumably a case of paraphrenia as described by Kraepelin. In any case there is nothing in his diaries or in the material afforded by his biographers to confirm his fantastic accounts regarding super-normal faculties, to say nothing of the claim of his divine mission.

There is, however, one intrinsic weakness in the usual psychiatric approach to cases of this class. The current system of clinical psychiatry failed to provide for the possibility that a person, besides suffering from a schizophrenic or paraphrenic psychosis, may in actual fact be subject to telepathic or "psychic" experiences. Indeed, it has failed to make allowance for such occurrences at all in either health or disease, and accordingly it is bound to turn a blind eye to their existence. We have discussed the reasons behind this attitude on an earlier page, and emphasised that, if maintained, it may seriously hamper the advance of science. But in no branch has this attitude been so detrimental as in the field of medical psychology. Not only does it prevent the proper appreciation of the mass of experimental evidence afforded by modern psychical research, but also of the telepathic aspects of such mental disorders as were discussed in the foregoing chapters. Little wonder that, accordingly, the claims of what in common parlance are now being described as *psychics* are being dismissed without a hearing, brushed aside as deliberate lies, or simply put down as additional evidence of mental disease which has to be classified alongside the rest of the delusions of a mental patient. It is clear that in these circumstances psychiatry had no reason to be anxious to find a proper niche within its system for persons exhibiting genuine psychic traits. It could safely go on denying their existence.

What, then, are the characteristics of the so-called psychics? Do they represent a characterological type of their own, and, if so, what is their correlation to other characterological types such as Kretschmer's schizoids and schizothymics? It may be as well to remark that we shall be able to discuss these questions in a tentative way only. The study of character requires detailed information on a person's life-history, of his family background, aided by prolonged observation and psychological analysis of his behaviour. But on attempting to apply this approach to the personality of an alleged psychic, we must first possess reliable data upon which his classification within this group can be based. These data are now forthcoming, thanks to the increasing volume of information afforded by modern psychical research. But as a general rule we look in vain for facts regarding the characterological aspects of the subject with whom the E.S.P. experiments are being carried out. Problems of character lie either outside the range of the experimenter's interest or he has to withhold relevant facts for reasons of privacy. In some cases he may have to couch whatever information he is able to gather in such terms as to make his report more of a conventional eulogy of Mr. X. or Mrs. Y. (to whom he is indebted for his or her ready co-operation, etc.) than an objective psychological statement. In any case, he can hardly risk describing his subject as a schizophrenic borderline case, a drug addict, a fraud, or a mixture of all the three, even though he may have good reason to think so. There are two cases only at my disposal in which I was able to surmount these difficulties. They may serve as a starting point for our discussion.

CASE I

The identity of our first subject can be revealed. It is Mrs. Eileen Garrett, the well-known English medium whose autobiography, entitled *My Life As a Search For the Meaning Of Mediumship*, contains a remarkably frank account of her personality in most aspects relevant to our issue. Indeed, her book can be classed as a valuable human document ranking alongside the confession of such Christian mystics as St. Teresa of Avila, or St. Catherine of Siena, or in a smaller way, of E. Swedenborg. But the chief significance of her case to our inquiry lies in the fact that besides her well-known record as a trance medium, Mrs. Garrett has been one of Dr. Rhine's successful percipients in E.S.P. experiments.

During her stay in the U.S.A. in 1934, he worked with her for three weeks and carried out a series of card-calling tests under various conditions, both in trance and in the waking state. In his *New Frontiers of the Mind*, Rhine reports that in spite of her dislike of laboratory conditions, Mrs. Garrett did extremely well under telepathic conditions and was in a class with that of his " very best " subjects. " Altogether, the work with Mrs. Garrett was among the most interesting we have done. Her averages, omitting a final week during which she was manifestly ill, were about 10.1 for telepathy in the waking state, and 9.1 in trance. In more than 8000 trials with clairvoyance she averaged only 5.7 correct hits in 25 trials in the waking state and 5.6 in trance. But even so, results with such a large number of trials are significant. During the high point in her curve, for a three-day period, she rose to an average of 6.3 in clairvoyance in 3500 runs and to 13.4 in telepathy."

A further group of tests was next designed to imitate more closely her usual work as a trance medium. Rhine describes how, in a series of sittings, it was arranged that persons unknown to Mrs. Garrett were brought to the laboratory " under carefully guarded conditions ", with a view to finding out whether information could be given that could not have been obtained by Mrs. Garrett by the normal methods of sense or of reason. To exclude the senses, the subject was brought into the room only after the medium was put into trance. " The subject was then seated behind her and was asked to remain silent throughout the sitting and to leave before the medium woke from trance in case there were other sittings with the same visitor." Stenographic records were taken of all that the medium said, and a special method of " matching ", devised by H. F. Saltmarsh and S. G. Soal, was applied to evaluate results. It was found that under these conditions " Mrs. Garrett produced knowledge unquestionably extra-sensory in origin in connection with various visiting subjects." Dr. Rhine adds that her work as a whole also passed the mathematical criterion of extra-chance results.

It is readily understood that no such standards can be applied to the rest of her mediumistic manifestations. They are of the same order as the productions of such high class mediums as Mrs. Willett or Mrs. Osborne Leonard to whom we referred in Chapter VII. But apart from her reputation with the general public their authenticity has been acknowledged by such an authority as Dr. William Brown. I have to add here in passing only that in 1938 S. G. Soal and K. M. Goldney tried to duplicate Dr. Rhine's card-calling tests with Mrs. Garrett this side of the ocean, but with negative results. Disappointing though this may be to a staunch advocate of the volitional nature of the E.S.P. faculty, it is fully consistent with our interpretation outlined in Chapter III, and does not detract from our interest in her case as a successful percipient.

What then, is the characterological background of Mrs. Garrett's psychic disposition?

To answer this question I propose to examine her autobiography: (*a*) from the psychiatric point of view, to analyse her account in the way of a case history supplied by a patient, taking nothing for granted and ready to class experiences which are at variance with our familiar concepts as symptoms of mental disease. However, it goes without saying that such an approach is bound to destroy all semblance of supernormality which may be suggested by her case, to dissipate her personal myth, as it were. I propose, therefore, to supplement this approach by discussing her account, (*b*) in the light of the telepathy hypothesis in order thus to arrive at a balanced picture of her personality as a whole.

(*a*) *Psychiatric Aspects*

Eileen Garrett started life under tragic circumstances: her mother, the youngest of a family of thirteen, came from straight-laced southern Irish Protestant stock but had married a Spanish Catholic of doubtful character. For this she was expelled from her family and she committed suicide soon after giving birth to her child. Six weeks after her mother's death, her father took his life by shooting himself. Eileen was brought up by an aunt in a farm-house near Dublin, and it appears from her account that her foster-mother lacked all understanding of the highly sensitive and imaginative child. Her uncle, more sympathetic, and perhaps more readily acceptable to her as a father-substitute, seems to have done little to allay her sense of frustration. Eileen grew up a lonely child and sought refuge in day-dreams and phantasies in the company of what she called her "Unseen Children", a boy and a girl, who came to visit her any time she cared. So firm was her conviction of the reality of these imaginary playmates that she was deeply shocked when her aunt questioned their existence. In the absence of real friends to play with, and real people on whom to lavish her affection, she got more and more entangled in her world of phantasies and grew increasingly resentful of her aunt. She describes how at the age of five or six she resorted to all sorts of mischievous pranks, acts of senseless destruction and cruelty. She would break pieces of china, tear pages out of a bible, etc., in order to challenge God in whom, in defiance to her aunt, she refused to believe. On one occasion she killed a whole brood of baby ducklings (her aunt's favourites), wondering how she would be punished and secretly hoping that the chastisement would be meted out by her uncle. In the further course, crows and little rabbits became the victims of her sadistic turns which were, however, followed by waves of remorse and an exalted feeling of sympathy with all suffering creatures. During all this time Eileen was given to wandering and truancy ; shy before strangers, seeking to avoid contact with the real world and preferring to be left alone to indulge in her phantasies.

Her relatives, realising that she was beyond their control, sent her to a boarding school at Dublin. But here, too, she was antagonistic to her teachers, and resentful of their lack of understanding for her idiosyncrasies.

She had a frail physique and her school attendance was broken by frequent ailments such as measles, bronchitis, whooping cough and pneumonia, but she was prematurely developed in sexual respects. At the age of thirteen she was involved with other girls in a nightly escapade, meeting boys from a nearby college. She was discovered and expelled from school.

On her return from the boarding school, her aunt revealed the tragic story of her parents, not concealing the fear that she might have inherited her mother's waywardness and headstrong nature. This disclosure only increased Eileen's resentment of the strict Protestant family tradition, her hatred of the aunt, and her rebellion against all those in authority. At fifteen, she was advised to be taken into the drier atmosphere of the South of England for reasons of health, and in the year that followed, she lived with relatives of her aunt in London, where her stay proved a success. She found she was no longer regarded as a boisterous girl in her 'teens, but a promising young woman whose air of eccentricity gave her a charm of her own.

At sixteen, she married a man much older than herself for whom, on her own admission, she did not really care, and it appears that she married him as a means of escape from continued dependence on her aunt.

She soon realised, however, that she had to pay dearly for

her freedom. " My honeymoon was a miserable experience. I found myself daily rebelling against the thing I had done and I would have made any sacrifice if I could have found some way of being relieved of my new relationship."

Growing disharmony between them arising from sexual difficulties was greatly aggravated by her habit of day-dreaming and " sensing and visioning " and resulted in her husband becoming increasingly concerned about her mental condition.

She reports in her book that her " Unseen Children " ceased visiting her when she reached the age of puberty. They were replaced by a wealth of other visions, no less vivid and colourful. From early childhood she had been in the habit of " seeing " not merely the physical bodies of people, but of noticing that each person was set " within a nebulous egg-shaped covering of its own. This surround as I call it for want of a better name, might consist of transparent changing colours or sometimes becoming dense and dull in character. The state of these coverings altered according to the variation in people's moods. . . . I knew that the character of people depended on their surrounds. By the quality of the light and colour they gave forth I could judge their personality. Some people moved in grey shadows and some in glowing lights. For me the important thing about anyone I met was to see and feel the quality of these surrounds." But these intriguing experiences were not confined to hallucinations of lights and colour only ; there were occasions when she was aware that the air was full of singing sounds and " globules of light " dancing like midget stars in space. Sometimes she would feel that she herself was drawn into their movements, or that she would split up " as though divided into little pieces, and each piece was located in a different place ". Or else she saw the conversation of people " shaped in space in flowing colours " and she would become aware of their thoughts " as forms of light moving towards their destiny, either dissipating or impacting, according to the force with which they had been projected ". On another page she describes a typical instance of so-called depersonalisation and loss of feeling of reality, associated with what textbooks of psychiatry term autoscopic hallucinations. " I was sitting one day in a chair in a quite relaxed and passive state, wondering whether I should get up, when looking ahead of me I saw a shadowy replica of myself." Later on she suddenly realised that she could see more easily and clearly " with her finger tips " or through the nape of her neck, than through her eyes, and " hearing came " to her through her feet and her knees. In that state she felt sound as an " external current entering her body from without and vibrating through its bony structure ". In these conditions she would be heard talking aloud to herself without knowing it or else she would develop an attack of nausea and " lightness in the head ".

Experiences like these seem to have become crystallisation points of what, in terms of clinical psychiatry, would be described as systematic delusions. " Studying the nature (of the surrounds) I became convinced that they had a positive and important function as a protection to what we call physical body. . . ." Another of its functions was that of an " All-discerning Eye which penetrated beyond man's ordinary vision ". Many pages of her autobiography are devoted to further elaborating this system in all earnestness.

However, Mrs. Garrett herself seems to realise that she was " surely heading for madness " at that time : moreover, her health was further undermined by three consecutive pregnancies. Her first two children died in infancy from meningitis, whilst her third baby survived only a few hours after birth. Several physicians were called in, a psychiatrist consulted and a blood test taken, of which we only learn that it was a negative. For obvious reasons Mrs. Garrett's account of this period is fragmentary. She writes with indignation of the psychiatrist's suggestion that the death of her children was due to inheritance of disease from herself, whilst her husband's sexual inadequacy was the probable cause of her " hallucinations ". She even goes so far as to make his diagnosis responsible for the final break-down of her marriage.

We do not learn the precise nature of the diagnosis suggested by the psychiatrist. But on the ground of Mrs. Garrett's account, it is easy to guess. There has been evidence of an eccentric disposition from early childhood. Her tendency to mental dissociation and day-dreaming, coupled with what her relatives regarded as fantastic lying must have been strongly suggestive of hysteria. So was the dramatic impersonation of her phantasies by what she called her " Unseen Children ". However, at a later stage, her hallucinations assumed an increasingly schizophrenic colouring, as illustrated by her " seeing " through her finger tips, or the nape of the neck. So-called extra-campine hallucinations of this kind are generally regarded as symptomatic of a serious mental disorder, and so are her systematised delusions, centred around the All-discerning Eye. Again, her attitude towards her aunt and her teachers had undoubtedly a slight paranoic colouring, whilst her claims to possess psychic or supernormal faculties may easily be regarded as symptoms of megalomania. The reported suicide of both her parents would then complete the picture of a schizophrenic or paraphrenic psychosis with ideas of grandeur in a constitutionally abnormal individual.

However, the diagnosis of a full-fledged mental disease was given the lie by the further development of Mrs. Garrett's personality. She soon regained her mental balance, took part in a successful business enterprise, first with a friend and, subsequently, on her own account. At the beginning of the Great War we see her running a restaurant and a Hostel for Officers in London. We see her getting her divorce from her first husband on the grounds of adultery on his part, marrying a second time and, following the death in action of her second husband, trying her luck in a third marriage. We also see her taking part in political life, joining the Fabian Society and pursuing a variety of other interests and activities in the years that followed.

The rest of Mrs. Garrett's life-history, fascinating though it be, shows little of interest from the psychiatric point of view. Apart from what she describes as the gradual development of her psychic faculties there is no more evidence of mental abnormalities. She gains considerable reputation as a trance medium, follows calls to the U.S.A., works with Dr. Rhine at Duke University and, on her return to England, with Dr. Soal and Mrs. Goldney. Finally, she returns to the U.S.A. where, at the age of nearly fifty, she establishes a successful publishing house of her own. Clearly, this is not the history of a schizophrenic patient, and even the diagnosis of a mild paraphrenic psychosis through which she passed following her first marriage would hardly cover all the aspects of her case. How, then, should it be assessed from the medico-psychological point of view?

(*b*) *Psychic Aspects*

Our tentative psychiatric appreciation of Mrs. Garrett's personality left many gaps in her life-history; we referred to most accounts of her "sensing and visioning" as to symptoms of mental disorder in the clinical sense, we treated them as evidence of hallucinations or delusions of grandeur and did not consider the possibility that there might be an element of truth in her claims. But the striking fact is that her autobiography is punctuated by numerous accounts of experiences, which to the student of psychical research, bear all the hall-marks of authenticity. She describes how, at the age of seven or eight, she had the vision of her favourite aunt Leon appearing to her in broad daylight, saying: "I must go away now and take the baby with me". Aunt Leon lived twenty miles away and Eileen did not know that she was expecting at that time, nor had she any notion of what pregnancy meant. On recounting to her aunt her strange experience she was reprimanded for having told a lie. But the next day her relatives received news that both aunt Leon and her newborn baby had died in point of fact the day before!

On another page Mrs. Garrett describes a similar experience she had soon after her second husband had left for the front. First, she felt that he was going through hours of "terrific suffering and fear", and goes on to say: "In order to relieve the strain of what I was feeling about him I gathered some friends together to go out to dine and dance. At 11.30, as I went out of the crowded room, the vision of my husband dying began to open; I seemed for a moment to have lost my own identity, and was caught in the midst of a terrible explosion. I saw this gentle, golden-haired man blown to pieces—I watched the pieces fall; I swam out of a sea of sound. When I came to myself I was sitting in the foyer of the restaurant alone. I knew that my husband was killed. . . . Two days later my husband was reported missing. A week later the official word came from the War Office that he was listed as dead."

We will recall here our old grievance that spontaneous

experiences of this kind have the drawback that they cannot as a rule be verified. However, we may also recall that Dr. Rhine's successful series of E.S.P. tests carried out with Mrs. Garrett may rightly be considered as collateral evidence of her psychic faculties and that an important aspect of her mediumistic productions was likewise verified under strict experimental conditions. All this gives added significance to her extraordinary experiences, although it may well be that the majority was derived from auto-psychic sources, and only a smaller part of hetero-psychic origin.

However this may be, the modern medico-psychological approach has shown increasing readiness to take the reports given by our patients seriously. Following this principle no psychiatrist would doubt Mrs. Garrett's account of her autoscopic or extra-campine hallucinations. Why, then, should we reject her stories of alleged telepathy "from the dying"? We accepted her phantasies of the "Unseen Children" as a true description of subjective experiences, originating from the auto-psychic sphere. Why should we stop at this point and discard all accounts pointing to the occasional emergence of similar experiences from the hetero-psychic sphere as deliberate lies? In short, why should we give credence to the psychiatric aspect of her case history only and refuse it to the psychic aspect? This is certainly not to suggest that we should take each and all of her claims at their face value. Clearly, our task must be to sift the available evidence from the angle of both the orthodox psychiatric and the telepathic points of view and to sort out the wheat from the chaff, figments from facts contained in her account.

It is interesting to trace back the gradual development of Mrs. Garrett's psychic trend into her years of childhood. She describes how as a girl of five or six she would seek refuge in her room in order to shake off her sense of being "too close" to other children. "I felt as a child hurt and oppressed by any close contact with others." In her view the protection gained in her solitude marked the beginning of her ability to "draw within" and live alone with herself. In the further course she learned to "withdraw" from the world without, fleeing into her room. During this condition of "withdrawal", she asserts she was safe from insult or injury by her enemies. "When I lived in this separated state no one was really able to reach me and they could no longer cause me either hurt or confusion. If this were madness then I had no more fear of it, because in this state alone was I truly peaceful and happy."

But she soon realised that these blissful states were often coupled with an increased influx of impressions from both the auto-psychic and hetero-psychic sphere. In the period which preceded her nervous break-down these experiences became more and more obtrusive. She complains of the "unbearable strain of being the unwilling recipient" of impressions of this kind. She now tries hard to prevent "this invasion of external happenings from tearing" her nervous system to pieces; she appeals to God to assist her in shutting out "the impact of these unwanted experiences". But her attitude towards them tends to vary from time to time.

At the beginning of her career as a trance medium she is either strangely elated, or deeply stirred, by the appearance of her trance controls *Uvani*, the Oriental youth, or *Abdul Latif*, the Persian physician. She expressly says that there seems to exist a hidden correlation between her ambiguous attitude towards suffering and pain and a similar attitude towards the trance state and all it meant to her. I may remark here in passing only that this ambivalent attitude is obviously conditioned by what psychoanalysts would call her unresolved Oedipus complex in relation to her aunt and her uncle, and that this may be partly responsible for the adult edition of her "Unseen Children". But whatever the reason, she remains divided in her mind regarding most aspects of her mediumship and her psychic gift in general. She is either inclined to refer to it as a supernatural endowment, as a means of spiritual enlightenment and mystic communion with the divinity, or else she is sorely aware of its morbid implications, of her urgent need for self-protection against what Jung called the Perils of the Soul, against the danger which her psychic disposition entailed to her mental balance and sanity.

It will be noted, however, that her reaction to the impact of hetero-psychic experiences never assumed the degree of frantic desperation or the dismal negativistic colouring characteristic of paranoic schizophrenia. At its worst it is confined to a transient spell which soon yields to a more placid and optimistic attitude towards the world. This became increasingly obvious in her later years. At the time of writing her biography she seems to have succeeded in putting her house in order, in reconciling the " normal " and the " supernormal " aspects of her life with each other and in bringing them under something like a unified command.

The reasons for this ultimately favourable course can only be guessed. One may be the absence of true paranoic features in Mrs. Garrett's mental make-up. Put in terms of the telepathy hypothesis this would mean that her " intuitions " did not, after all, run along the one-way track of the paranoic reaction type, that her hetero-psychic sensitiveness referred to other things than the repressed aggressive tendencies of her fellow-men. This is illustrated by two episodes in her life-history. She recounts that the last straw which led to the break-down of her first marriage was her husband's adultery with another woman. Far from " sensing " this state of affairs telepathically, she learned of it in a roundabout way and seems to have been rather taken aback by the news. The second example is less striking, but equally significant. Dr. Soal and Mrs. Goldney, trying to duplicate Rhine's E.S.P. experiments with Mrs. Garrett, had arrived at a negative result and did not conceal their disappointment in their subsequent publication. However, Mrs. Garrett, utterly unaware of her failure, dictates to Mrs. Goldney a description of her own reactions, full of optimism about her work with Dr. Soal which, she feels, is more likely " to bring out her mediumistic capabilities than would the Duke conditions ",—that is, the experiments with Dr. Rhine.

Clearly, this is not the reserved, suspicious attitude of a paranoid or schizoid personality. It is the genial approach of a woman, impassive to implied criticism, yet easily suggestible and influenced by persons stronger than herself. It has obviously been a similar approach to people, to private and business affairs in general, which accounts for both her failures and successes in life. Although it is difficult to assess whether and how far her intuitive gifts were of greater assistance to her in other cases than in the two instances just described, they can certainly be exonerated from the charge of having twisted her outlook in such an ominous way as we are wont to see in the paranoic reaction type. Indeed, a biologically more congruous trend of the underlying hetero-psychic sensitiveness, however fallible, seems to be a fundamental characteristic of the psychic temperament. In the chapter that follows I propose to examine a second case of this type.

Chapter XII

PORTRAIT OF A "PSYCHIC", CASE 2

THE identity of our second case—we may call him Mr. Scott—cannot be revealed. He is one of the most successful percipients in the Duke type of E.S.P. experiments and worked particularly well under telepathic conditions. Details of the experimental results which would give clues to his identity are irrelevant to our present issue ; be it sufficient to say that he maintained highly significant extra-chance scores over a period of years under conditions equalling the very best achieved by Rhine and his associates. I had the opportunity of meeting him during his short stay in this country and my interview with him was witnessed by some members of the Council of the Society for Psychical Research to whom I have to express my thanks for their co-operation. My wife, who took notes of our conversation, was also present.

For obvious reasons I am not in a position to present a complete case history of Mr. Scott, and I had also to refrain from physical examination. However, he was fully aware of the objective of our meeting and answered all my questions readily. Scott is a gifted cartoonist, aged forty-one. He was born in the Southern States of the U.S.A., has been married for seven years but is separated from his wife. They have no children. He is of asthenic habitus and states that he is suffering from cardio-vascular disability for which he was recently released from the U.S. Army. He reports that during the past years he has been in the habit of taking a fair amount of alcohol. Our conversation began at about 4 p.m. during which I noticed his face was slightly flushed and that he was obviously under the influence of a moderate amount of drink.

Scott had been brought up under unhappy family conditions, and frankly stated his father was a drinker. " I am like my father, you know . . .", he said. " He was soft and emotional and so am I. He liked drink and so do I. I am just like my father."

Scott was the second of a family of six. One brother—two years his senior—lives in South America, his four sisters "somewhere in the States". He never got on well with Bill and there was frequent friction between them. One of his early recollections is of his father giving one of his sisters a "bad hiding". For all he knew no one in the family had anything like psychic gifts, although one of his mother's sisters who died in childhood, despite being mentally defective, was something like a child-prodigy and could speak several languages fluently.

Scott states that he first became aware of his psychic powers by his "magic" influence over other people, particularly women. He was able to attract them to himself through the powers of his mind. These powers made themselves felt also in various other ways. It often occurred to him that he would paralyse people just by looking at them: for instance, when they tried to pick a quarrel with him he would simply stun his attacker with his eyes, "perhaps it is hypnosis". One night, someone started an argument with him in a night-club. Without touching him he threw him down the stairs. He thought it was not quite fair to use his powers in such a way. Years ago he said that he noticed that he possessed the gift of being able to ward off death from a dying person by holding his hand or by stroking his forehead. He gave a somewhat rambling account of several instances in which this happened; all of them utterly unconvincing.

Mr. Scott further states that, besides being able to influence other people mentally, he is himself exceedingly sensitive to the thoughts of his fellows. He claims that he gets a picture of their personalities "in a flash", often accompanied by a vague impression of colour. "Colour", he exclaims, "is the great thing. Black and White give you a flat, two-dimensional notion of things; colour provides the third dimension." This is what he intuitively senses in his fellow men. It tells him whether they are good or bad, friendly or hostile towards him. "Of course, it is often far from pleasant. Sometimes I enter a pub and I feel: this fellow is going to start a fight with you. I can't bear his looks. . . . Or is it that he can't bear *mine?*

Sometimes I need not even see his face. I can feel his look from behind. It may make me so uneasy that I must leave the place."

He was less communicative when our conversation turned to his married life. "I am now getting my divorce from my wife. We are the best of friends, but we simply cannot get on with each other any longer. We are getting on each other's nerves. I am too sensitive to what is going on in her mind. Sometimes my intuition makes life intolerable to me—and to the people who have to live with me." He impulsively turned to my wife and grasped her hand: "You see, I feel that you are deep, very deep indeed . . . there is something encouraging in you, something that you convey without talking."

At certain points of our conversation, Scott seemed to strike a visionary note. He would lower his voice and remark enigmatically: "There is something religious about these psychic powers. I often feel they are something heavenly; something from another world." He intimates that they may in fact have been bestowed on him directly from God, although he hesitates to say so expressly. Another of Mr. Scott's claims refers to the gifts of prophecy. Our conversation took place in the winter of 1943, and he remarked with emphasis: "Great things are going to happen soon. Perhaps invasion this month. The war will end October next. But, to be sure, it will first have to run its full course." (I have to insert here that a few months back, at the time of Mr. Roosevelt's journey to meet Mr. Churchill, he had predicted that the President would never return and would be killed at sea. Yet his friends assured me that Scott was undismayed by the persistent failure of his prophecies to come true. Nothing seemed to shake his conviction of his infallibility.)

He appeared obviously flattered by the interest which was now being taken in him by the medical profession. He spoke incessantly, frequently changing his subject, unable to focus his attention for any length of time. Sometimes he would break off in the middle of a sentence, walk up and down the room, light a cigarette on the wrong end, throw it away, take another one and do the same thing all over again. Or he would summon us to a bare wall in order to illustrate his point by an imaginary picture on the wallpaper. The picture was meant to convey three things in a surrealistic manner: the Sun, a Beam of Light and the Sword. The Sun, he said, is the Lord God, the Beam of Light is God's influence upon mankind which he, Scott, was destined to convey to the world through his art. "You don't just draw pictures of things, it should always be Light that is made visible by the artist. That is his mission."

I have to add here that despite his eccentric behaviour, Scott has always contrived to make a good adjustment to the requirements of ordinary life. I learned from friends who have known him for years that in addition to his work as a cartoonist and a poster designer he was running a small business of his own and had always shown good common sense in his transactions.

At the time of writing, two years after the interview described here, Scott has remained the same eccentric as before without evidence of mental deterioration. He is still successful in his business affairs and his health has improved. His attitude towards his psychic gifts seems to have somewhat changed and he appears to be disappointed by his failure to utilise his "intuition" in making money at horse races or games of fortune. He has been less ready to co-operate in E.S.P. experiments. Neither was he willing to see me again at a second visit which brought him to this country from abroad. In other respects he has not altered. He maintained his conviction of his infallible psychic powers, his belief in his "higher" mission, as well as his convivial habits and his liking of drink.

1. *Psychiatric Aspects*

This is as far as the information goes which is available in our second case. Taken at its face value, it is undoubtedly suggestive of mental disorder. I described Scott's eccentric behaviour, his lack of concentration, the wandering of his associations, his tendency to think in symbols rather than in clear-cut concepts, his failure to appreciate the inconsistency of some of his statements, his claims to be able to hypnotise an opponent into submission, to be irresistible to women by dint of his psychic faculties and, last but not least, his veiled intimation to his higher mission. All this is gravely suspicious of delusions of grandeur. Again, his impression of colour when looking at people may be interpreted as a hallucination or pseudo-hallucination of the kind described by Mrs. Garrett.

On the other hand, there is evidence of vague ideas of reference and persecution in his statements. He enters a room and knows at once that one of those present is going to pick a quarrel with him. He senses that an "evil eye" is fixed on him behind his back and he expressly says that sometimes he may be hard put to it to ward off such sinister influences. In a similar vein, his guarded references to his matrimonial difficulties show striking resemblance to Strindberg's complaints of his agonising sensitiveness to the variations of his wife's feelings towards him, quoted in Chapter VIII.

Statements like these have an unmistakably paranoic colouring and can well be taken as additional confirmation of a delusional trend existing in a constitutionally eccentric individual. However, here again, as in the case of Eileen Garrett, it would be obviously wrong to class Scott as a mental patient in the orthodox psychiatric sense. In the first place, we have to make allowance for his slightly alcoholic condition during our conversation. We know that this alone may suffice to bring out certain features suggestive of mental disorder (although it is equally true that chronic alcoholism may itself be an important conditioning factor for the development of paranoic psychoses in persons with a primarily schizothymic disposition). A more cogent argument against the diagnosis of a full-fledged mental disorder in Scott's case lies in the fact that, apart from his matrimonial difficulties, he has been able to maintain ordinary relations with his fellows, to look after his business interests, to manage his own affairs, in short, to avoid certification, which, as my teacher Professor Wagner-Jauregg once put it, is the only valid criterion of a person's sanity.

Again, from the characterological point of view it is obvious that Scott does not fit in with the familiar picture of the schizothymic or schizoid type of personality. We described him as a "good sport", as a lively conversationalist, a man easy to approach and to influence, quick in forming friendships and with an apparent flair for the sympathetic understanding of other people. For instance, his impulsive remark to my wife in which he tried to sum up her personality seemed to hit the nail on the head. It lends colour to his claim to " see " the characters of other people " in a flash ", to assess them in what is usually described as an intuitive way. All this goes far to show that, like Mrs. Eileen Garrett, Scott's personality could more appropriately be described in terms of a *psychic* than a schizothymic temperament.

2. *Psychic Aspects*

I emphasised that whatever be our verdict of Scott's case, whether we class him as a psychic, as a borderline schizophrenic or paraphrenic, there is a vast mass of experimental evidence available which shows him as a highly successful percipient in E.S.P. tests under telepathic conditions. I also mentioned that his tendency to extra-chance scores was maintained for a number of years so that it cannot possibly be attributed to a temporary E.S.P. phase only, but to a trait intrinsic to his personal make-up.

This gains added significance when we recall our tentative telepathic interpretation of the paranoic reaction type. I pointed out that part of the patient's paranoic trend may be due to sensitiveness to hetero-psychic material of a particular sadistic-aggressive kind, and that at a later stage the gradual deterioration of his personality may be associated with a gradual increase of his range of telepathic sensitiveness. We saw that, on the other hand, hetero-psychic sensitiveness may cover a wide variety of mental processes, thoughts, emotional attitudes, etc., without undue emphasis on sadistic-aggressive tendencies. This point was illustrated by what we described as Mrs. Eileen Garrett's genuinely psychic trend. In Mr. Scott's case the paranoic element is obviously more in evidence, but certainly not to such a degree as to stamp him as a paranoic or paranoid schizophrenic. Moreover, we have seen that his whole characterological make-up differs from the familiar schizothymic temperament. We stressed his free and easy manner, his good contact with and his sympathetic understanding of his fellow-men, we pointed to his marked suggestibility. Indeed, it may well be asked whether his psychiatric appreciation as outlined above was not itself influenced by his susceptibility, telepathic or otherwise, to unconscious preconceptions and expectations of my own. I called attention to such a possibility on an earlier page and pointed out that it may vitiate the outcome not only of experiments in telepathy, but of practically all kinds of psychological investigations. It may be as well, therefore, to reconsider the psychiatric interpretation of his case from this point of view, that is to say, in the light of what I called the hypothesis of telepathic leakage.

I saw Scott at a time when I was engaged in the first formulation of my theory of paranoia and paranoic schizophrenia, expounded in the third part of this book. On recalling the argument there pursued, the reader may be struck by the far-reaching correspondence between some of Scott's references to his " Mesmeric " powers and my own thesis. Indeed, this is so unmistakable that it may well be asked whether I did not fall the victim of my own unconscious suggestions which were being reflected by the patient. But if this were the case, it would only illustrate my point and lend colour to the statement that, as a true psychic, Scott is sensitive to influences which are at bottom of telepathic nature. Indeed, it would suggest that Scott, in unwittingly reproducing part of my own emotionally coloured mental contents only confirmed my views, much in the same manner as did Mesmer's somnambulists, Charcot's hysterics or some of the patients subjected to more up-to-date methods of psychotherapy with regard to the views held by their respective physicians or analysts.

However, there is an important point of difference. Whilst the possibility of telepathic leakage did not occur to Mesmer, Charcot or to the protagonists of the modern schools of medical psychology, it lies at the root of our conception of the "psychic". I pointed out that it is a fundamental feature of the psychic temperament to respond to thoughts and expectations in the minds of their fellows, to assume, like chameleons, the colours of the surrounding objects and to reflect them as if they were their own. This has obviously happened during my interview with Scott, also to my mental picture of the psychic type of personality, derived as it was from my previous acquaintance with similar types. But far from falsifying the principal characteristics of the portrait outlined here, it only throws one of its essential features into sharper perspective.

To avoid misrepresentations, I may add one point. There can be no doubt that, notwithstanding Scott's chameleon-like suggestibility, he was genuinely eccentric to the core and that his portrait, as depicted here, squares with the impression he gave to his friends and relations. I may also mention that prior to my examination he was interviewed by a noted American psychiatrist and that his diagnosis was in far-reaching agreement with my own, at least as far as the psychiatric aspects are concerned. My American colleague, too, classed him as a border-line case with marked schizoid features, perhaps on the verge of a schizophrenic psychosis.

Indeed there is little doubt that the paranoic element is more pronounced in his case than in the case of Eileen Garrett, whereas hysteric features are much less in evidence in his make-up. But this is again in good keeping with our interpretation. There obviously exist all shades and grades of transition between frankly paranoid and psychic personalities, with a varying admixture of hysteric traits. On the other hand, the fundamental difference between the two types has become abundantly clear from our considerations. The paranoic patient, and to a lesser degree, the schizoid and schizothymic type, is sensitive to repressed sadistic-aggressive tendencies in the minds of his fellows. He taps a remote and, as a rule, more or less inaccessible, level of their unconsciousness. By contrast, the psychic is sensitive to a different pattern of psychological processes, predominantly located in the preconscious sphere and of a biologically less incongruous character. More often than not, his reactions may be vitiated by what we described as telepathic scatter, but sometimes they may strike us as genuinely intuitive, or " supernormal ". This has quite obviously been the case with regard to the E.S.P. experiments carried out with both Mrs. Garrett and Mr. Scott, and in a less conclusive manner, with regard to the mediumistic work of the former. On the other hand, we have seen that Mrs. Garrett's early history, as well as some of her trance productions, showed evidence of a marked hysteric involvement, while Mr. Scott's personality exhibited features of a paranoid disposition.

All this goes far to show that, as a matter of principle, the psychic type of character may contain traits which overlap with both the schizothymic and the hysteric temperament, though it is identical with neither of them. It represents a characterological type of its own, marked by a special susceptibility to hetero-psychic influences, a susceptibility which may either remain latent and manifest itself in occasional psychic experiences only, or which may be so pronounced as to bring the person concerned right on the verge of mental disorder.

It is readily understood that here, again, we may find an infinite variety of transitional types between the full-grown picture of the psychic and the "normal" characterological make-up. We may have such morbid geniuses as Emanuel Swedenborg and August Strindberg at one end of the scale and at the other such unassuming cases as the patients whose telepathic dreams we described in Chapter V. There may be

> Conquerors and Kings
> among them
> Founders of sects and systems, to whom add
> Sophists, Bards, Statesmen, all unquiet things,
> Which stir so strongly the soul's secret springs,
> And are themselves the fools to those they fool.

of whom Byron sang in *Child Harold's Pilgrimage.* There may be men of profound culture and creative genius, sensitive to unfathomed depths of the human mind, poets of the stature of William Blake, Wordsworth or Walt Whitman; writers of such eminence as Dostoevsky or Proust, scholars of such distinction as Professor Gilbert Murray, and many others who may themselves remain largely unaware of their latent psychic propensities; and there may be, finally, the man in the street (very often it is a woman) who has barely more than an intuitive flair for the personalities of his fellows which, for all practical intents and purposes, may be difficult to distinguish from ordinary common sense, based on experience and a subtle gift of observation.

It must remain an open question whether there is a correlation between such cases of pronounced mental disorder as are found at the morbid end of our scale and the clinical picture of paraphrenia expansiva or phantastica as described by Kraepelin. Clearly, this problem cannot be decided on the basis of such fragmentary evidence as is available at present. It rather raises further questions which call for investigation. Are psychics in general more prone to paraphrenic disorders than other people? Conversely, do some (or possibly all?) paraphrenics whom we meet in mental hospitals exhibit traits of a psychic disposition, or have they at least passed through a psychic phase? And what is the correlation between the psychic type of character and so-called spiritualistic psychoses? These questions open up a fascinating field of psychiatric research towards which the two cases reviewed here cannot make more than a tentative contribution. But tentative though it be, it shows that a future scientific approach to the problem of the psychic type of character will have to be based on two things. First, on an approach to our ordinary clinical material with an open mind, ready to accept the challenge of facts which have so far been out of bounds to the clinical psychiatrist and, secondly, on a proper appreciation of the modern E.S.P. tests and their statistical evaluation, on which, in the last resort, the exact diagnosis of the psychic predisposition—as outlined here—has to rely.

Chapter XIII

PERSONALITY RESTATED

"Supreme goal of human striving thou art personality."—GOETHE.

AN inquiry of the kind pursued here must inevitably come to grips with the problem of personality. Telepathy may be described as immediate awareness by a person of another person's mind. But if this is possible one may well ask: where does the boundary line of one person's mind end and the mind of the other person begin? We located the sum total of a person's mental processes, conscious, pre-conscious, and unconscious, into the auto-psychic sphere and said that telepathic experiences are derived from the hetero-psychic sphere. But how does the occasional short circuit between the two spheres come about, or rather, what is it that makes such an event the exception and not the rule? In short, what constitutes the frontiers of personality in the light of the telepathy hypothesis and what are the safeguards which insure its continued existence in the face of the possible intrusion of hetero-psychic experiences into an individual mind?

Evidently, these questions touch upon problems which go far beyond the scope of our present inquiry. Like Time and Space they are problems which fall into the domain of the philosopher whose job it will be to reconcile his basic propositions with the newly established facts of psychical research. In the present chapter we shall be content to give in barest outline our ideas on how the facts we have discussed affect the current psychological concept of personality and leave to a future date the filling-in of details and the bearing our conclusions have upon the views held by other students of medical psychology and psychical research.

However, we cannot further elaborate our thesis without at least a tentative statement of the correlation which exists between what we described as the auto-psychic and the hetero-psychic spheres to Freud's concepts of the unconscious, the Ego and the Super-ego. The reader, familiar with the elements of Freud's doctrine, will realise that despite departures (which to the orthodox follower may appear little short of blasphemy) the argument presented here is based on certain fundamental presuppositions of psychoanalysis. There is, in the first place, Freud's topographical conception of the mind falling into an unconscious, pre-conscious and a conscious part. There is, secondly, his dynamic conception of the inter-relationship between these three departments, of the forces which are responsible for shutting out a substantial part of psychic processes from the conscious sphere, or else for their occasional intrusion into consciousness under the symbolic guise of dreams, neurotic symptoms or faulty actions. There is, thirdly, Freud's economic interpretation of the working of this intricate machinery in terms of the pleasure-pain principle, that is to say, as a machinery operated by the lust for gratification of wishes and desires, sexual or otherwise, and by the anxiety to avoid pain and discomfort.

This is but an incomplete summary of the principal tenets of psychoanalysis such as have become common ground to modern medical psychology. But it will be noted that, within limitations, they have served as a satisfactory basis for most of our formulations. However, I pointed out in Chapter VI that there is no room left for telepathy and related phenomena in the system of orthodox psychoanalysis and that, worse still, it has failed to make allowance for their very possibility. Accordingly, it has remained, to say the least, indifferent to the occurrence of telepathy in the psychoanalytic situation, to what I described as telepathic leakage and, consequently, to the risk that it may vitiate some of its basic principles. I also stated that to make amends for this shortcoming of the analytical doctrine would require its revision and re-statement from the angle of psychical research—a formidable task for which the time has obviously not yet come. But focussing attention on broadest outlines only, it appears that the appreciation of the very existence of telepathy from the psychoanalytical point of view requires little more than an expansion of Freud's original topographic formulation of the mind beyond its narrower confines. This we have done when we suggested that, if certain conditions are fulfilled, hetero-psychic influence from the pre-conscious or unconscious of another person may intrude into our consciousness, much in the same way as this may occur to unconscious or pre-conscious material of our own. In fact we intimated that this process is subject to the identical laws of symbolic representation as was described by Freud with regard to so-called primary mental processes. Lastly, we stated, that hetero-psychic elements seeking to intrude into the auto-psychic sphere may meet with the same forces of censorship, resistance or repression which are operative in shutting our pre-conscious or unconscious material from our consciousness.

This is as far as we could go in reconciling facts revealed by our inquiry with certain basic presuppositions of psychoanalysis. How, then, do our findings affect the Freudian picture of the Ego, and what may be called the classical conception of personality in general? It may be as well to state outright that Freud's formulation, ingenious though it be, in mapping out the conscious, pre-conscious and unconscious sections of the Ego, in describing the gradual development of the Super-ego, etc., fails to give a satisfactory explanation of the problem of personality as a whole. Freud shows how the machinery works, how it pursues its purpose to seek pleasure, to avoid pain, but he cannot account for the ultimate determining factor that sets the whole machinery going and gives it the semblance of a purposeful, self-willed and, at bottom, transcendental psychological entity.

Freud compares this entity with a horseman riding a horse who may hold that it is he who decides upon the course of his ride, whereas in reality he only yields to the primitive urges and desires which stir the horse under him. However, Freud's simile begs the issue. The fact that a good horseman is able to master his horse can only be denied if we take the absence of his free will for granted, whatever be its philosophical implications. It has been rightly stated that this weakness of Freud's theory is at bottom intrinsic to the essentially mechanistic, causal approach of psychoanalysis, and that Adler's essentially teleological doctrine, inquiring as it does into ends instead of into causes, brings into focus a more significant aspect of the self.

The problem, put in this way, seems to lead us on the

treacherous ground of metaphysical speculation. However, we shall presently see that it is not therefore necessary to refer the case of Freud's melancholy horseman from the medical psychologist back to the Philosophical Out Patients' Department. This is in any case little likely to offer a more satisfactory solution of his problem than was forthcoming since the days of Plato, Descartes, Leibnitz or Hegel. I propose to show that our interpretation of the attitudes assumed by the sceptic who denies telepathy; by the paranoic patient who struggles against it; and by the psychic who may readily yield to its appeal, give at least a tentative clue as to the factors which are involved in the emergence of personality in the psychological sense, even though we cannot venture to deal with the philosophical and, in the last outcome, transcendental aspects of the question.

We pointed out that the scientist and the educated public, anxious to maintain their unconditionally rationalistic outlook, may choose to deny facts which seem to endanger their beliefs. Modern man has evolved his scientific world picture on the ruins of the magic and animistic creed, in defiance of its secret appeal to the primitive forces in his own mind. He tries hard to prevent the Return of the Repressed into his ordinary experience. In his iconoclastic zeal he has destroyed all the pagan gods which survived in the temple of modern science and snubs anyone daring to assert their continued existence, or worse still, trying to retrace the outlines of a faded archaic image, or to piece together the fragments of a broken sacramental figure which once adorned the altar of primitive man. He seems still to be afraid that the monstrous idols of a past epoch may be raised on to the place which they once occupied and become the objects of outrageous worship.

It is obviously this overzealous rationalism which accounts for the scorn and ridicule which is still being meted out in certain quarters to those engaged in the new research. I pointed out that in some respects it is strangely reminiscent of the attitude which academic psychology had assumed towards psychoanalysis in the early days. Indeed, Freud himself has shown that this reaction was nothing else than a manifestation of resistance on a vast scale against some of the less palatable sexual implications of his teachings. However, it will be noted that what we here described as the Return of the Repressed is of an altogether different order from Freud's original conception of repressed mental contents. Repression in the sense applied here is more readily comparable with the gradual elimination in the course of evolution of characteristics with what biologists termed negative survival value, such as the hypertrophic body size of certain antediluvian reptiles, or the tendency to walk on all fours in our own racial past. Paul Schilder referred to this process as organic repression, claiming for it a wider connotation than for repression in the orthodox Freudian sense. However this may be, the force of repression—organic or otherwise—directed against the return of magic and animistic ways of thinking is an unmistakable feature of modern man's bias against telepathy and related phenomena, whatever the reasons that account for it.

The frantic attempts of the paranoic and catatonic patient to ward off the return of the repressed in his own mind throws some of these reasons into sharper perspective. In his case it is no longer the merely academic consideration of such a possibility that arouses his apprehension. The unspeakable has actually taken place. It did not occur to him in his dreams and phantasies only, it overtook him in broad daylight, shaking the very foundation of his existence, breaking the sheet-anchor of his sanity. In Chapter IX I described in greater detail the successive phases of his struggle with the " renegade forces of his soul ". I showed how at a later phase of the process he may be overwhelmed by the maddening influx of hetero-psychic influences into his consciousness, how the frontiers separating his mind from other individuals (and from the outer world in general) may be gradually abolished, leading to the terminal stage of schizophrenic deterioration and to the final disintegration of his personality.

Again, in describing the characterological type of the psychic, we saw that at one time or another he, too, may go through a psychotic phase, closely resembling true schizophrenic reactions. In other cases, we stated, he may pass into states of mystic illumination in which he feels that his personality dissolves itself into a " boundless being ", in which " death was an almost laughable impossibility—the loss of personality seeming no extinction, but the only true life "

(Tennyson). Numerous passages conveying the same idea could be quoted from the writings of medieval saints and mystics as well as from the works of nineteenth-century romanticism.

The bearing of these observations upon the problem of personality is obvious. They lay open the roots of modern man's profoundly suspicious attitude towards the "super-normal" aspect of his existence. Modern man is anxious to maintain his control over the irrational undercurrents of his mind. He is determined to prevent the "Return of the Repressed" into his consciousness. He instinctively feels that his overthrow in the silent struggle with what Jung called the *Perils of his Soul* might endanger his sanity and spell the doom of his personal existence, even though his physical health and bodily integrity might remain unscathed. But our observations show at the same time that there is an ingrained tendency in our mental make-up which militates against the intrusion of hetero-psychic influences into our mind, a psychological diaphragm whose business it is to prevent the occurrence of telepathy and which subjects such hetero-psychic material as may penetrate through the diaphragm to much the same forces of repression as were described by Freud. Whatever be the metaphysical nature of personality, there can be little doubt that the tendency just described is one of the essential pre-requisites of its existence. Its failure to maintain its protective screen entails mental derangement. Its complete break-down leads to the break-down of the personality, whilst a transient permeability of the screen to certain patterns of psychological processes may lead to such occasional telepathic occurrences as we have seen during casual absent-mindedness or in states of minor emotional disturbance.

Personality thus conceived is not a final and undisputed achievement. It is the resultant from two apparently irreconcilable antagonisms such as are inherent in all natural phenomena. It is a dynamic principle concerned with the isolation of a self-contained psychological entity from the rest of the world, and safeguarding its unity and coherence in the dimensions of both space and time; it is like the crest of a wave thrown up by the ocean for a split second of individual existence before it falls back into the sea.

It might be objected here that this formulation, derived as it is from observations in the field of abnormal psychology and psychiatry, meets only the case of certain morbid aspects of personality and fails to give a reasonable account of its "normal" features. However, it is interesting to note the striking correspondence of our thesis with the idea held by a number of modern thinkers who approached the problem from an entirely different angle. I need only mention the Russian philosopher Nicolas Berdiaev. Berdiaev likewise holds that the achievement of personality is the fruit of an "heroic struggle"; that its realisation is accompanied by pain and suffering and that its self-fulfilment is the *summum bonum* of human life. Such pathological conditions as we discussed in the foregoing chapters only accentuate this state of affairs. The schizoid or schizothymic type of character is more anxious to maintain his personality because it is exposed to greater dangers than the personality of any other characterological type. Such aberrations of personality structure as are found in psychics and hysterics illustrates the same point. Indeed, it may well be that the best way of arriving at an understanding of the normal structure of personality lies in the proper appreciation of its functioning under abnormal conditions. It will be noted that the medical man, called upon to give a definition of physical health, may resort to much the same expedient.

However this may be, our interpretation of the problem of personality is in a much better position to account for the newly established facts of psychical research than most of the older "classical" concepts. On laying the finishing touches to the manuscript of this chapter I find that Whately Carington, in his recent book on *Telepathy* attacked the same problem from a different angle. Whilst I have the greatest admiration for his work I think that his association theory of telepathy shows its principal weakness precisely in regard to his treatment of personality. In Carington's view the human mind consists of an aggregate of sensa or images, so-called psychons, which are linked together by the laws of association. But on denying the reality of a force which is responsible for their coherence, personality dissolves itself in thin air, or is at least reduced to a shadowy existence with no conceivable boundary lines to make it a clearly discernible island in the midst of the uncharted sea of a mysterious World Mind.

* * * * * * *

But the interpretation suggested here throws light not only on the dynamic principle which is operative in the maintenance of the mature personality and in its protection against the *Return of the Repressed* from both the auto-psychic and hetero-psychic sphere. It also enables us to give a tentative description of certain developmental aspects of personality. There is a consensus of opinion that the new-born infant can hardly be regarded as a personality in the psychological sense. It is little more than a bundle of reflexes, automatically responding to what environmental influences it is subjected to. His body is equally strange to him as the objects of the outer world, they merge into one another much in the same way as in the case of a deteriorated schizophrenic. When he begins to talk his speech echoes what he hears from his parents and nurses ; it does not, for the first two or three years, contain the momentous word *I*. One could say that both mentally and physically he remains part and parcel of his begetters, that his psychological segregation from his mother lags behind his biological segregation from her organism ; that despite the fact of his physical birth he seems still to be connected with her through something like a psychological umbilical cord.

Only by degrees does he reach the stage of a self-contained personal existence and more often than not he has to do so against the unconscious opposition of a strangely possessive maternal instinct. The fact is that there exists a natural tendency on his mother's part to identify herself with her offspring in a literal sense, to regard him as flesh and bone of her own, to consider his bodily functions as the functions of her own body, to maintain control of his feeding habits, of the actions of his bowels and bladder as if they were operated through her own will, as if they had remained her direct and exclusive responsibility. But unless there is a hitch in the ordinary course of events the growing child soon arrives at the stage when he refuses to be merely the passive object of maternal care and solicitude. He responds to stimuli of the outer world in his own way ; he seeks to avoid pain and to gain pleasure from his experiences on his own account; he fights for an existence independent of the will of his parents and nurses. He may decide to take or refuse food after his own liking; he may insist upon emptying his bladder or his bowels at times of his own choice. He may set his claim for a truly individual existence against the tendency inherent in many parents to expand their own range of personality by jealously clinging to their hold over the personalities of their own children.

Psychoanalysts have been well aware of this fact and described the secret struggle which forms an undercurrent of the familiar child-parent relationship as manifestations of the so-called Oedipus complex, giving it largely sexual interpretation. Seen from our angle, this struggle assumes a different complexion. It is the struggle for the final emancipation of the child's self from the parental mind, an expression of the prolonged birth-labours of the emergent personality, of the individual in the making.

But in the course of the third or fourth year this process is usually completed. By that time the child has severed the last delicate fibres—the primitive animal tie—as Anna Freud put it—that connected him with the motherly roots of his life. He has attained full command of language, he is able to speak of himself in the first person and to voice his protest against excessive parental solicitude if need be. On the other hand, it is obvious that he is still readily accessible to the moulding influences, to the continuous suggestions, direct and indirect, verbal and non-verbal, which emanate from his parents and educators. This is the time when the so-called introjection of the father's or mother's images into the child's ego is taking place, when their authority is being embodied, as it were, into his personality, a process described by Freud as the formation of the Super-ego. It is at the same time the first attempt of society to gain control over the self-seeking interests, over the untrammelled urges and desires of a recalcitrant outsider. It will be noted that our description of this development runs along parallel lines with those drawn by Adler and his school. It will also be recalled that in our view it is largely the way in which the individual grapples with the tasks of his self-assertion and the preservation of his personality, as opposed to the claims of the outer world, which ultimately determines the development of his special characterological type.

But we intimated that children usually retain a natural susceptibility to hetero-psychic experiences and such an authority as Dr. C. D. Broad has pointed out that this may account for much of the normal child's ability to learn, to respond to guidance, for his intuitive understanding of the minds of his parents and teachers. Here again, observations under pathological conditions seem to lend colour to this point. A significant example is the case of Ilga K. to whom we referred on an earlier page ; more recently a number of similar observations in mentally defective children, though much less spectacular, have come to my notice. Another interesting example are neuroses which can be observed in children of neurotic parents or in neurotic family situations in general. Such cases may be largely due to common inheritance or to adverse environmental conditions obtaining in the family, but in a group of observations described by psychoanalysts the part played by what we described as telepathic leakage is unmistakable.

I may quote the case of Rita, aged three, contained in Melanie Klein's book, *The Psycho-analysis of Children.* Rita was suffering from an obsessional neurosis which seemed to duplicate most of the symptoms of a similar neurosis found in her mother, including its hidden sexual implications. The same refers to Ruth, aged four, whose analysis was carried out with her older sister present who had in turn been undergoing psychoanalytical treatment. Melanie Klein's patient, Peter, aged three, was likewise suffering from a neurosis with all the paraphernalia of sexual symbolism of adult type. He, too, had been brought up in thoroughly neurotic family conditions. But the striking fact is that, apart from such symptoms as might reasonably be attributed to inheritance or adverse environmental influences, these children seemed to exhibit knowledge of sexual matters far in excess of what could be expected at their age and of which, more often than not, the ordinary citizen only learns from reading Melanie Klein's books. Still, there is not the slightest reason to doubt the *bona fides* of her report or of similar accounts presented by other child psychologists. However, whilst psychoanalysts may be satisfied with the explanation that such knowledge is derived from unconscious sources, from something like a racial memory in which Jung's archetypes or primordial images have been preserved, here, again, it is obvious that observations like these can just as well be attributed to such hetero-psychic influences from the analyst upon the patient as we discussed in Chapter VII, reinforced by the special susceptibility of children to such influences.

This is also illustrated by John Layard's account of the Lady of the Hare to whom we have briefly referred before. In this case the analyst subjected the mother of a feeble-minded sixteen-year old girl to psychological treatment and he reports that while the analysis of the mother made satisfactory progress the mental condition of her daughter, too, seemed to improve. Shy and inhibited before, she became more sociable and more amenable to discipline. Layard claims that this effect is nothing but a striking manifestation of a direct intercommunication, as it were, between the mother's and the child's unconscious.

However, in the course of the gradual development and consolidation of the personality of the growing child this susceptibility to telepathy and related influences recedes more and more into the background. It may be confined to a few isolated occurrences only, such as were described in earlier chapters, or else it may only be preserved in a special characterological type, in the type of the psychics. The gradual consolidation of the dynamic personality structure is only broken by the profound neuro-glandular changes that take place in puberty. This seems to entail a temporary loosening of the texture of the screen which safeguards the integrity of the self, and this is obviously the reason for some of the striking psychological manifestations of the puberty period. It is the time when the young man and woman find themselves first confronted with the problem of sex, coupled as it is with the challenge to renounce once again the " splendid " isolation of their personalities so anxiously guarded, though offering them in return the priceless award of companionship, the bond of love and affection to restore their communion with human society which they lost when the last fibres connecting them with the minds of their parents were torn. We know that the reaction of the individual to this challenge (and this chance) is ambiguous. It may manifest itself in the familiar self-consciousness and shyness of the adolescent boy or girl, sometimes bordering on paranoic conditions. Alternatively, it may lead to highly coloured sentimental moods, to states of exaltation, to experiences reminiscent of mystic ecstasies or may even usher in true schizophrenic psychoses.

However, once the adolescent has passed through the critical phase of puberty he has usually reached the stage of final consolidation of his personality structure. In primitive societies this is acknowledged through special initiation rites following which a lad is accepted as a member of the tribe, admitted to its councils and given a share of common rights and responsibilities. He ceases, once and for all, to be nothing but an offspring of the personalities of his begetters. He receives the formal approval of society to live a life of his own, as a self-contained individual, subject only to the anonymous forces of what Gustave Le Bon, Wilfred Trotter and McDougall described as the Crowd, the Herd, or the Group Mind, which seek to maintain their sway over him.

Whether and how far a telepathic factor is involved in these influences is a highly controversial matter. More recently Dr. L. Bendit and Whately Carington called attention to the claims of Marais and Fabre that such termite communities as the bee-hive or the ant-heap behave much in the same way as human crowds or mobs under certain conditions. Some authors have gone so far as to suggest that their collective behaviour may be directly controlled through influences of an extra-sensory nature and that the same may be true for the human counterpart of the termite community: the totalitarian state. Freud put forward a similar suggestion and pointed out that telepathy may be nothing else than "the original archaic method by which individuals understand one another, and which has been pushed into the background in the course of phylogenetic development by the better method of communication by means of signs apprehended by the sense organs".

However, statements like these are largely a matter of conjecture at the present state of our information and modern biologists are not prepared to acknowledge the existence of a group-mind as an independent, supra-personal psychological entity. If this is true we must consider human personality as a unique achievement in nature, perhaps closely approximated by the higher mammals, yet unrivalled on the plane of collective animal behaviour or human group formation. Obviously, the modern pattern of society is built on an entirely different principle, to the exclusion of telepathy as a factor to knit together its members in a higher order of social organisation. It is based on the co-operation of men and women on the *rational* plane, on their readiness to subordinate their individual aims and ambitions to common needs, on their ability to plan their lives and their social systems undeflected by irrational undercurrents of their minds.

Certainly, this is a largely Utopian picture of society, and mankind will have to go a long way to put it into practice. But there can be little doubt from what we have said about the intrinsic trend of human personality that the development of mankind tends towards growing consolidation and integration of the dynamic personality structure, as opposed to its merging into a mysterious, supra-personal World Mind. This is expressed by the line from Goethe which I quoted at the beginning of this chapter. It has been an omen of fateful significance that his maxim of personality as the " supreme prize of human striving " has been thrown by the board by the German nation. At the time of writing the concluding chapter of this book, history has already spoken its verdict of a people—and of its leaders—who have chosen to regress to an atavistic form of social organisation, to relapse to obsolete patterns of behaviour and experience, characteristic of the insect state. To those who are able to grasp its meaning, the sign-post of Evolution points in the opposite direction.

CONCLUSIONS

WHAT then, is the part played by telepathy in man's mental organisation?

Is it a newly evolving faculty which would enhance the depth and width of our vision far beyond the boundaries of ordinary human experience, as Frederic Myers asserted; "a first faltering intimation of a new thrust forward on the part of a purposive life force", as Dr. Joad put it? Or is it a developmental throw-back as was assumed by Freud and Henri Bergson, a vestigial function of the human mind to which it has recourse whenever the "attention to life" is in abeyance? Is it a power stretching forward to the angels, or is it going back to the amoeba as was suggested by Professor Thouless?

Most of the evidence reviewed here tends to confirm the latter view. We defined telepathy as awareness by a person of another person's mental state without the aid of the usual channels of sensation. But this awareness is dim and uncertain, subject to errors of refraction, as it were, caused by the vagaries of the unconscious strata of the mind through which it has to pass. It does not convey the picture of real things, it is confined to indirect, symbolic representations of ideas, or images, like the dream or the neurotic symptom. It slips from the essential to the accidental, from the agent's central idea to an association which is only remotely connected with it. We described this tendency as a tendency to deviation in the associative sphere and emphasised that precisely the same tendency may be responsible for such temporal dislocation or displacement of telepathic scores as has been found by Whately Carington, Soal-Goldney and others under experimental conditions.

There is no use denying that so-called pre-cognitive and post-cognitive reactions of this kind enhance still further the impression of intrinsic improbability created by the phenomena, that is to say: their inconsistency with what Thouless described as our established system of scientific expectations based on long experience. But once the initial difficulties of revising this system of expectations in the light of an additional body of experience are surmounted, the fact of spatio-temporal dislocation or *telepathic scatter* loses much of its paradoxical character and only throws the primitive vestigial nature of telepathy into sharper perspective. It suggests that, apart from giving a distorted picture of processes in another person's mind, telepathy is also apt to reflect them with utter disregard of their temporal order. It may present them either *after* the actual event, suggesting the existence of a latency period, or *ahead of time*, giving the semblance of prophetic anticipation.

It is readily understood, however, that such reactions, no matter how striking they may appear, are totally undesirable from the biological point of view. Thouless illustrated the point by describing the embarrassment of a deer that would have to rely on its telepathic, or clairvoyant ability to make it aware of the danger of a tiger. It would be unable to decide whether this danger referred to a tiger in the vicinity now, to one a hundred and fifty miles away, or to one that would be there to-morrow. And to this we have to add that if it were a deer conversant with the subtleties of Freudian symbolism it could not even be sure whether the animal was a tiger at all and not a veiled intimation of sexual aggression.

All this goes far to show that nature had good reasons to suppress what tendency there may be in the animal kingdom to the development of telepathy and related phenomena. In this respect the succour it receives from the negativistic attitude of many respectable academic psychologists and psychiatrists towards them cannot be but highly commendable. Indeed, we have seen in the chapters dealing with the psychiatric aspects of our problem that the shutting out of hetero-psychic experiences from our minds is one of the essential pre-requisites of our sanity. We also pointed out that alternatively, a lesser degree of impairment of the protective screen in our mind to prevent their intrusion may lead to minor abnormalities only of character.

It is against this background that the question of deliberate cultivation of paranormal cognition must be considered. On the ground of the available experimental evidence this possibility cannot be denied. Rhine and his followers have succeeded without doubt in bringing about an atmosphere in which a large number of subjects produces remarkable records of extra-chance scores. But it should not be overlooked that these successes were only attained on the level of statistical significance and never reached the standard of biological expediency. They might pass Dr. R. A. Fisher's x^2 test of chance probability, but they would certainly fail when put to the test of everyday life. Even Rhine's champion percipients were unable to guess every card every time with anything like the accuracy required from ordinary sensory functions. Obviously, the inherent tendency to telepathic scatter rendered them unable to do so.

On the other hand, it would be rash to assert that telepathy and related phenomena are nothing but morbid and biologically unwanted features of the human mind. We intimated that the primary susceptibility of the child to hetero-psychic experiences may be responsible for the intuitive background of his orientation in the world, and we emphasised that apart from such characterological border-line cases as pronounced psychics, perfectly normal and well-balanced individuals may preserve a similar approach to their fellow-men in adult age. In Western civilisation this seems to be the prerogative of a certain highly sensitive artistic type, to which we have to add the comparatively harmless specimen of anti-intellectualist philosophers and less harmless intuitive political leaders. But it appears that they are more widespread in oriental peoples and, indeed, constitute an integral part of the ancient Indian and Chinese mentality.

Striking a balance between the credit and debit side of psi-phenomena there is, after all, little to commend attempts at their systematic development outside conditions of the laboratory experiment. The way of the mystic who turns a blind eye to the real world in order to open his senses to the experience of the Unseen World, is not the way of modern man. In prehistoric times, and in certain epochs of recorded history, it may have yielded powerful impulses to human betterment; it may have enriched the spiritual landscape of man and made him aware of problems beyond the immediate grasp of his reason. But experience has shown that it is inconsistent with the tasks of everyday life and with the general trend of contemporary civilisation, which cannot afford to be run by methods of trial and error, characteristic of the mystic outlook. Intuition may suffice to span the gulf between the problems of this world and the World Hereafter ; it may succeed in devising systems of thought to satisfy what Schopenhauer called man's metaphysical needs, but it cannot be expected to build bridges safe enough to carry the weight of a calculated volume of traffic, or to master the wealth of administrative, technical and economic problems of modern society upon which the health and happiness of ordinary men, women and children are based.

Indeed, history to-day has led to a definite cleavage on this score and proved the ascendancy of a truly rational approach to the world, as opposed to the non-rational approach of a past age. But this precisely makes a dispassionate inquiry into the latter aspect of our mind more imperative than ever before, however reluctant we may be to acknowledge its very existence. Freud has pointed out that man's objective in life should be to make the Unconscious conscious. To this we may add the challenge of making the Irrational rational by tackling it with modern methods of research, psychical, psychological or otherwise.

This is one of the conclusions at which we arrive from our reading of the problem of telepathy. It is closely allied with conclusions which suggest themselves in a field more directly concerned with medical psychology.

The telepathy hypothesis gave us a key to a new understanding of the structure and development of personality, and thus helped to throw fresh light on various problems of abnormal psychology and psychiatry. It led to a new interpretation of the paranoic reaction type and schizophrenic deterioration, and to the conception of the psychic type of character as a counterpart of Kretschmer's schizothymic and cyclothymic types. But the significance of telepathic phenomena as conceived here is not confined to their implied warning that : " That way madness lies ". We intimated that they may play an important part in the psychoanalytical situation and necessitate a revision and re-statement of some of the basic propositions of psychoanalysis. It can well be expected that this may in turn open up new prospects of psychological treatment. Obviously, hetero-psychic experiences are not only a potential source of danger to our psychological equilibrium ; they can just as well serve as vehicles for our therapeutic suggestions. Indeed, we hinted that what we described as telepathic leakage may not only be responsible for the origin of some of the mutual contradictions of the rival schools of psychotherapy, but may also account for some of their therapeutic achievements.

It is true that influences of this kind are essentially uncontrollable and therefore inconsistent with a rational scheme of treatment. But our newly gained information may prove to be of value to our psychotherapeutic approach in another way. It may assist in imparting to the patient a more detached attitude towards such morbid symptoms as are due to heteropsychic influences. This may be helpful in early paranoics and schizophrenics, or following shock or convulsion therapy in more advanced cases. Dr. L. Bendit, in his book on *Paranormal Cognition*, and John Layard, in his *Lady of the Hare*, quote promising instances of psychotherapy moving along these lines. In a similar vein a new approach to the treatment of problem children and behaviour problems in adolescents may be opened up through fresh insight gained into what we described as the dynamic structure of personality and our interpretation of the child-parent relationship.

However, it need not be emphasised that it would be premature to expect therapeutic results, ready for application in everyday practice, from an approach to medical psychology which has barely got beyond the stage of assembling its facts and stating its first principles. Moreover, we have to admit that our present information about an important aspect of paranormal cognition, namely, its physiological basis, is more than incomplete. We are able to give a description of the psychological conditioning factors of telepathy, to tabulate the laws which it obeys, but we cannot tell in what way the phenomena come about ; we know of no anatomical substratum to account for their origin, and still less are we able to explain their apparent action at a distance in flagrant contradiction to the familiar radiation laws.

However, if it is true to say that there is an unbridgeable gap in our knowledge of the *modus operandi* of telepathy and related phenomena, it may be as well to realise that a similar rift can be discovered running through all the branches of contemporary psychology, if only we are prepared to see it.

Dr. Thouless pointed out that the essential characteristic of the scientific type of explanation is that " one thing can only cause another if there were a continuous chain of physical events between the two ". He illustrates this point by an example taken from the field of visual perception and describes how electro-magnetic waves come from the object to the eye, produce chemical changes in the retina, travel along the optic nerve to the visual area of the brain cortex, etc., and he adds : " If we *ignore* * the problem of how a material change in the cerebral cortex is related to the conscious process of perception, and confine ourselves to the physical process between the emission of rays from a material object and the completion of a muscular, or glandular response on the part of the organism, the continuity of the chain of physical processes is complete ".

But it is obvious that disregarding the gap which exists between the chain of physical processes described and the conscious appreciation of a sense impression is merely a matter of scientific expediency. We have become used to glossing over its existence because we cannot help it, and because we found that it is possible to build up a working system of psychology even though we are incapable of filling the gap ; indeed, the success of the behaviourist school of psychology has shown that the study of human behaviour can go a long way without any reference to its existence.

What, then, do we learn from this state of affairs ?

In what way does it help to reduce the alleged intrinsic improbability of the phenomena and to reconcile them with our familiar body of experience ?

We described telepathy as perception by one person of another person's mental processes, as what we called hetero-psychic awareness, and contrasted it with the awareness by a person of his own mental processes, that is to say, of his auto-psychic experiences. We were able to show, furthermore, that experiences from the hetero-psychic sphere are subject to much the same psychological forces of repression and resistance and to the identical laws of symbolic representation, distortion and condensation, as experiences emerging from pre-conscious, or unconscious strata of the auto-psychic sphere. It is true that we are unable to say in what way hetero-psychic awareness

* The italics are mine.

comes about. But the fact is that we are equally unable to account for the last stretch of the way in which auto-psychic experiences are being registered in our minds.

To put it in other words, there is a far-reaching similarity between auto-psychic and hetero-psychic awareness, not only as far as their *modus operandi*, but also as far as the difficulty of their appreciation in strictly physical terms is concerned. The gap seems to be insignificant in the case of our ordinary psychological experience ; it appears to be disproportionately large in the case of alleged paranormal cognition, but it is essentially of the same order in both cases. The two are at the bottom of the same nature. The observations discussed here are not in reality inconsistent with established facts of our psychic life.

However, we have to make two qualifications to this statement : I pointed out in the previous chapter that the very fact of the existence of telepathy and related phenomena made a revision and restatement of the classical concept of personality necessary. I emphasised that in the light of the newly established facts the notion of human personality, as a strictly isolated psychic entity, can no longer be maintained, and seems to merge into the common pool of an all-encompassing Collective Unconsciousness, such as was visualised by C. G. Jung. But whilst Jung's conception was largely based on an assumed solidarity of the human species in the perspective of time, knit together by something like mental inheritance, our proposition (and similar views held by Tyrrell, Bendit, Carington and many others) implies the contiguity of the collective unconscious in the perspective of space, as it were, with no conceivable organic link to account for its origin. We already pointed to this difficulty by our reference to the gap within our recognised system of scientific expectations. But it reminds us once more that telepathy, and all it stands for, can only be reconciled with our familiar world picture at the price of throwing some of our cherished concepts of a strictly individual cerebral localisation of mental processes and perhaps of causality within the field of psychology in general, overboard.

The second qualification is necessary in view of the deliberate simplification of the argument pursued here. I pointed out in the preface to the book that I propose to confine considerations to the problem of telepathy pure and simple, and to leave the broader issues of paranormal cognition or psi-phenomena outside our frame of reference. However, a student of psychical research may rightly object there that telepathy is neither pure nor simple and cannot, in reality, be separated from clairvoyance, psychometry, psycho-kinetic effects, and the like. Such an objection would, indeed, be justified. But we have it on the authority of Dr. Rhine that the psychological conditions of E.S.P. are largely identical under telepathic pre-cognitive, post-cognitive and even clairvoyant conditions. Accordingly, we have good reason to assume that, *mutatis mutandis*, most of our generalisations may be valid with regard to a wider field of the phenomena, or at least, that their psychological interpretation may be possible by means of the same principles as outlined here.

But here again, it would be useless to deny the inevitable repercussions of the wider issues involved in our problems upon adjacent fields of science and philosophy. We were at some pains in the course of our argument to keep to our original time-table and to avoid trespassing upon ground outside the confines of medical psychology. Even so, we were unable to evade at some point or other guarded references to the classical concepts of Time and Space, inasmuch as they are affected by our findings. However, it cannot be the task of a first reconnaissance into the psychological No Man's Land reviewed here to enter into serious discussion of these problems. They are herewith respectfully passed to the philosopher who will have to say the last word—or at least write the next book about them.

BIBLIOGRAPHY

Medical Psychology

Adler, Alfred. The Practice and Theory of Individual Psychology (1924).
Baynes, H. G. The Mythology of the Soul (1940).
Bendit, L. Paranormal Cognition (1944).
Bleuler, E. Textbook of Psychiatry (1924).
Brown, W. Psychology and Psychotherapy (1940).
Burlingham, D. (Quoted from Freud).
Deutsch, Helen. Occult Manifestations during Psychoanalysis. Imago (1926).
Ehrenwald, J. Ueber das "Lesen" mit Umgehung des optischen Wahrnehmungs-apparates (Befunde in einem Falle von reiner Wortblindheit) *Zeitschr. f. d. ges. Neur. u. Psychiatr.*, 132 (1930).
Hirnpathologische Bemerkungen zu einem Falle von "paranormalen" Erscheiningen bei einem Kinde (F. v. Neureiter). *Ibid.*, 157 (1937).
Psychological Aspects of Telepathy. *Proc. Soc. Psych. Res.*, 46 (1940).
Telepathy in Macbeth? *Journal Soc. Psych. Res.*, 32 (1941).
Telepathy in Dreams. *Brit. Journ. Med. Psychol.*, 19 (1942).
Telepathy in the Psychoanalytic Situation. *Brit. Journ. Med. Psychol.*, 20 (1944).
Freud, A. and Burlingham, D. Young Children in War-Time. London (1942).
Freud, S. The Interpretation of Dreams (1913).
Totem and Taboo (1918).
Psychoanalytische Bemerkungen ueber einen autobiographisch beschriebenen Fall von Paraznoia (Dementia paranoides). Collected Papers. Vienna (1925).
New Series of Introductory Lectures on Psychoanalysis (1933).
Ferenczi, S. Contributions to Psychoanalysis (1916).
Fodor, N. Telepathy in Dreams. American Imago (1942).
Glover, E. Technique of Psychoanalysis (1940).
Hitschmann, H. Telepathy and Psychoanalysis. Imago (1923).
Hoch, A. Constitutional Factors in Dementia Praecox. *Review of Neur. and Psychiatry* (1910).
Hollós, J. Imago, 19 (1933).
Hinsie and Schatzky. Psychiatric Dictionary (1940).
Jackson, H. Evolution and Dissolution of the Nervous System. Selected Writings (1940).
Jung, C. G. Contributions to Analytical Psychology (1928).
The Integration of Personality (1940).
Psychology of Occult Phenomena. Sittings with S. W.
Klein, M. The psychoanalysis of Children (1932).
Kraepelin, E. Psychiatrie. 8th Edition, Leipzig.

Kretschmer, E. Physique and Character (1936).
Layard, J. The Lady of the Hare (1944).
Maudsley, H. Natural Causes and Supernatural Seeming (1939).
Millais Culpin. Spiritualism and the New Psychology (1920).
Mitchell, T. W. Medical Psychology and Psychical Research (1922).
Meyer, A. Fundamental Concepts of Dementia Praecox. *Br. M. Journ.* (1906).
Money Kyrle, R. Superstition and Society (1933).
Neureiter, F. v. Wissen um Fremdes Wissen, etc., Gotha (1935).
Prinzhorn, H. Psychotherapy (1932).
Róheim, G. Animism, Magic and the Divine King, New York (1930).
Servadio, S. Imago, 21 (1935).
Squire, P. C. The Clairpsychism of Strindberg. *Psychoanal. Review,* 29 (1942).
Stekel, W. Die Sprache des Traumes (1911).
Schilder, P. Imago, 20 (1934).
Sterba, R. Psychiatry, 4 (1941).
Storch, A. The Primitive Archaic Forms of inner Experience and Thought in Schizophrenics. Nervous and Mental Disease Monograph Series (1924).
Trotter, W. Instincts of the Herd in Peace and War (1916).
Weygandt, W. Der Occultismus, seine Grundlagen and Gefahren. *Arch. ges. Psych. und Neur.* (1939).

Psychical Research

Balfour, Rt. Hon. G. W. The Ear of Dionysios, etc. *Proc. Soc. Psychic. Res.* (1917).
Bergson, H. Presidential Address. *Proc. Soc. Psychic. Res.*, 27 (1915).
Carington, Whately. Telepathy, An Outline of its Facts, Theory and Implications (1945); American edition, Thought Transference: An Outline of Facts, Theory and Implications of Telepathy (1946).
Experiments on the Paranormal Cognition of Drawings. *Proc. Soc. Psych. Res.*, 46 (1940), etc.
Garrett, E. My life as a Search for the Meaning of Mediumship (1939).
Gurney, E., Myers, F. W. H., and Podmore, F. Phantasms of the Living (1886).
Hall, M. Radclyffe and Troubridge (Una). On a Series of Sittings with Mrs. Osborne Leonard (1919).
Kerner, J. The Seeress of Provorst (1845).
Myers, F. W. H. Human Personality and its Survival of Bodily Death (1920).
Price, H. 50 Years of Psychic Research (1939).
Richmond, K. *Proc. Soc. Psychic. Res.*, 44 (1936).
Rhine, J. B. Extra-Sensory Perception (1935).
Rhine, J. B. and Associates. Extra-Sensory Perception after 60 Years (1940).
New Frontiers of the Mind (1938).

SIDGWICK, H. Report on Further Experiments in Thought Transference carried out by Professor Gilbert Murray. *Proc. Soc. Psychic. Res.*, 24 (1924).
SINCLAIR, U. Mental Radio (1930).
SOAL, S. G. Fresh Light on Card Guessing. *Proc. Soc. Psychic. Res.*, 46 (1940).
and GOLDNEY, K. M. *Proc. Soc. Psychic. Res.*, 47 (1943).
THOULESS, R. H. Experiments on Paranormal Guessing. *Brit. Journ. Psychol.*, 33 (1942).
An Experiment in Symbolism. Paper read to the S.P.R., Feb. 1945.
TYRRELL, G. N. M. Science and Psychical Phenomena (1938).
WARCOLLIER, R. Experiments in Telepathy (1939).

GENERAL

BERDIAEV, N. Solitude and Society (1938).
BERGSON, H. Creative Evolution (1911).
BROAD, C. D. The Mind and its Place in Nature (1937).
BURNE, Ch. S. Scraps of English Folklore. *Folk Lore*, 20, p. 223.
CLEUGH, M. F. Time (1937).
DUNNE, J. W. An Experiment with Time (1929).
FRAZER, J. The Golden Bough. I. The Magic Art (1890).
FABRE, J. H. Wonders of Instinct.
LÉVY BRUHL. La Mentalité Primitive (1912).
The Primitives and the Supernatural.
MALINOVSKI, B. The Argonauts of the Western Pacific.
The Sexual Life of the Savages (1929).
McDOUGALL, W. An Outline of Abnormal Psychology. The Group Mind (1926).
MARAIS, P. The Soul of the White Ant.
MEGROZ, R. L. The Dream World (1939).
MURPHY, G. *Proc. Amer. Soc. Psychic. Res.*, 39 (1945).
READ, CARVETH. Man and his Superstitions (1925).
SOLLAS, W. J. Ancient Hunters and their Modern Representatives.
SUTTON, E. A. The Living Thought of Swedenborg (1944).
TREVELLYAN. Folklore and Folk Stories of Wales, p. 238 (1909).
TYLOR, E. B. Primitive Culture (1903).
WHITEHEAD, A. N. Science and the Modern World (1943).
WORCESTER, B. The Life and Mission of Emmanuel Swedenborg (1907).

GLOSSARY

Alexia, congenital : Inability to learn to read with the rapidity and skill which would be expected from the individual's achievements in other subjects.

Auto-psyche : The mind of oneself.

Agent : In tests for telepathy, the person whose mental states are to be apprehended by the percipient.

Association Test : A psychological test in which the experimenter calls out a word or shows a picture to the test-person, and the test-person is expected immediately to reply with the next association that comes into his mind.

Clairvoyance : Extra-sensory perception of objective events as distinguished from telepathic perception of the mental or subjective events of another person.

Catatonia : A subdivision of dementia praecox or schizophrenia.

Collective Unconscious : Part of the mind which, on the view of C. G. Jung, does not originate from personal acquisitions but in the inherited possibility of psychic functioning.

Complex : A group of emotionally invested ideas, partially or entirely repressed (E. Jones).

Cyclothymia : Mild fluctuations of the manic-depressive type that almost have the stamp of normal mood shifts.

Dementia Praecox : Old term used for Schizophrenia.

Depersonalisation : Loss of the sense of reality of oneself; a symptom of neurosis or mental disorder.

Dissociation : The segregation of a group of mental processes, separated off from consciousness.

Disintegration : Disorganisation of psychic processes, characteristic of advanced cases of schizophrenia.

Extracampine Hallucination : Hallucinations localised outside the sensory field.

E.S.P. (*Extra-sensory Perception*) *:* Response to an external event (perception) not presented to any known sense.

Hetero-Psyche : Another person's mind.

Irrational : In the present context used to denote something outside the province of reason, not contrary to it.

Medium : A person subject to mental dissociation amounting to trance states which are claimed to favour the origin of psychic phenomena.

Negativism : Negative attitude or behaviour.

Paranoia : Form of mental disorder presenting delusions of persecution of a well-defined type.

Paranoid : Relating to paranoia, resembling paranoia.

Paraphrenia : Term introduced by Kraepelin, closely related to paranoia, marked by phantastic ideas of grandeur with exaltation. Paraphrenia expansiva : seen only in women. There is no marked tendency to deterioration.

Precognitive Telepathy : Foreknowledge of something that will be known to the agent in a short time (Thouless).

Projection : Process of throwing out upon another the ideas or impulses that belong to oneself.

Psychic : characterised by being susceptible to psychic or spiritual influences. Persons prone to telepathy or related experiences.

Psycho-kinetic Effect : The direct influence exerted on a physical system by a subject without any known intermediate energy or instrumentation.

Psi-Phenomena : Term introduced by Dr. Thouless to designate telepathy, precognition and clairvoyance without implying a theory as to their nature.

Repression : The active process of keeping out and ejecting, banishing from consciousness, the ideas or impulses that are unacceptable to it.

Rorschach Test : A psychological test consisting of inkblots of various shapes and colours shown to the subject with the request to interpret them.

Sadism : The destructive instinct directed outwards, thereby acquiring the character of aggression. (Freud).

Scatter Theory : A theory suggesting that the tendency of telepathic guesses to slip from the conscious into the preconscious or unconscious sphere, as well as their tendency to temporal displacement, is due to the biologically incongruous character of telepathy.

Schizophrenia : A form of mental disorder characterised by a tendency to "split mind" and gradual deterioration of the personality. Often associated with delusions of persecution. Synonymous with dementia praecox.

Schizoid : Schizophrenic border-line condition, not amounting to schizophrenia.

Schizothymia : A normal characterological type with schizoid features.

Subject : The person who is experimented upon. Most commonly the percipient in E.S.P., though also the agent in telepathy.

Symbolic Representation : Conveying a psychic component by changing its content but preserving its pattern.

Telepathy : Awareness by a person of another person's mental contents without the aid of sensory channels. Extrasensory perception of the mental activities of another person. It does not include the clairvoyant perception of objective events.

Most definitions of medico-psychological terms contained in this Glossary are quoted from Hinsie and Shatzky (1940) Psychiatric Dictionary.

Definitions of technical terms used in the literature of psychical research are quoted from a Glossary appended to numbers of *The Journal of Parapsychology*, Duke University Press, Durham, N.C., edited by J. B. Rhine and Associates. The responsibility of the formulation of such expressions as Auto-psychic and Hetero-psychic experiences, the Scatter Theory and the Psychic type of personality is my own.

INDEX

For Product Safety Concerns and Information please contact our EU representative GPSR@taylorandfrancis.com Taylor & Francis Verlag GmbH, Kaufingerstraße 24, 80331 München, Germany

Batch number: 10725869

Printed by Printforce, the Netherlands